Danielle Collins' FACE Yoga

FIRMING FACIAL EXERCISES & INSPIRING TIPS TO GLOW, INSIDE & OUT

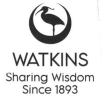

WATKINS
Sharing Wisdom
Since 1893

T0027095

Danielle Collins' Face Yoga

Danielle Collins

Dedicated to my family and friends
who inspire me every day.

First published in the UK and USA in 2019 by
Watkins, an imprint of Watkins Media Limited
Unit 11, Shepperton House
83–93 Shepperton Road
London N1 3DF

enquiries@watkinspublishing.com

Typeset in Brandon Grotesque and Walbaum
Colour reproduction by XY Digital
Printed in China

ISBN: 978-1-78678-245-8

Commissioning Editor: Kate Fox
Managing Editor: Daniel Hurst
Editor: Sophie Elletson
Managing Designer: Francesca Corsini
Production: Uzma Taj
Commissioned photography: Matt Lincoln
and Christina Wilson

A CIP record for this book is available from
the British Library

10

Publisher's note: The material contained in
this book is set out in good faith for general
guidance and no liability can be accepted
for loss or expense incurred in relying on
the information given. In particular this
book is not intended to replace expert
medical or psychiatric advice. This book is
for informational purposes only and is for
your own personal use and guidance. It is
not intended to diagnose, treat, or act as a
substitute for professional medical advice.
The author is not a medical practitioner nor
a counsellor, and professional advice should
be sought if desired before embarking on any
health-related programme.

www.watkinspublishing.com

Introduction   4

YOU AND YOUR SKIN   12

FACE YOGA AND YOU   36

FOREHEAD   80

EYES   90

CHEEKS   98

MOUTH   108

JAW   118

NECK   128

BEAUTY LIES WITHIN   138

A Final Word   168

INTRODUCTION

The Danielle Collins Face Yoga Method is a natural and practical way of looking and feeling healthy, happy, glowing and youthful. At its core, it is a combination of face exercises and massage, acupressure and relaxation techniques that are designed to lift, firm, smooth and relax the face and improve your overall wellbeing. This book will teach you how, why and when to practise Face Yoga and give you all the tools you need to implement these techniques in your everyday life.

MY WISH FOR YOU

I wholeheartedly believe you deserve to look and feel the very best version of yourself. My wish for you is that Face Yoga starts your journey to accept and love who you are, whilst simultaneously giving you a toolbox of simple yet effective techniques to look and feel even better.

In the coming chapters you will learn how to best use this book in your daily life, how Face Yoga works and how to live a healthy lifestyle to compliment this.

MY JOURNEY TO FACE YOGA

It was my 22nd birthday and for the previous few weeks, I had been planning my party. However, I couldn't even walk, let alone put on my party dress. My mind was blurred, my body fatigued and my arms and legs were consumed with unbearable aching pains.

A series of blood tests showed that I had been suffering from glandular fever and although it looked liked the end of the virus, it had left me with myalgic encephalopathy (ME), also known as post viral fatigue syndrome (PVFS) or chronic fatigue syndrome (CFS).

Over the next ten months my symptoms worsened. My muscles and glands hurt so much I often found it hard to walk from the bed to the toilet. My head felt like it was covered in a hazy fog and I found it hard to hold a conversation for more than five minutes.

I had to leave my job and stop exercising. My social life was non existent. Giving up everything that I loved felt like a kind of bereavement. Aspects of my personality changed too. I found that my confidence was lower than normal and I dreaded meeting new people.

Nine months into the illness I was referred to an ME specialist. He said that there was no single remedy to overcome ME but sometimes people found gradually building up activity and a combination of natural therapies like yoga provided some relief. After that appointment I decided I couldn't live like this any longer and was determined to find a way to nurse myself back to health.

NATURAL CURES

I spent time reading books, studies and magazines on natural health and ME. Gradually I started to put together an action plan of lifestyle changes I could make to rehabilitate myself.

Every day I practised five minutes of yoga. I discovered how to breathe correctly to calm my nervous system, boost my immune system and detox my body. My brain fog and my stress gradually started to reduce.

My research taught me that I had to transform my diet in order to overcome ME. I discovered sugar, caffeine and alcohol were impairing my immune system and depleting me of vitamins and minerals.

A NEW START

As I reached my 23rd birthday, my health started to improve. The muscle pain reduced, my head felt clearer, my energy levels were higher and I was able to do a couple of hours of activity a day. I felt it was time to think about the future.

Previous to my illness I had wanted to be a primary school teacher but I now felt that I was destined to use my experience of ME to help others. I enrolled in a diploma in professional relaxation therapy, which led to training as a yoga teacher and nutritional therapist, as well as training in face massage and pre- and postnatal yoga and introductory training in Indian head massage, the Alexander technique, Shiatsu and Thai Yoga massage.

When I was well enough to work again I started by teaching just one relaxation class per week. Then I built up to teaching individuals and groups yoga, wellbeing and nutrition. I also did wellbeing coaching for people with ME and I have been delighted to be able to help them in the same way I helped myself. Then, Face Yoga happened.

MY FACE YOGA METHOD

Early in my yoga career, I noticed how pleased my clients were with their results and remember one client saying to me, "I just wish my face matched my body". This echoed my own thoughts. I often wondered why we only trained in yoga techniques below the neck. There are so many muscles above the collarbone and these are the ones that are constantly on show!

FACE YOGA WORLDWIDE

The Danielle Collins Face Yoga Method was born from a combination of my training and many years of research. It is now enjoyed by millions of people worldwide through my videos, classes and courses. I have taught all over the world and appeared in hundreds of magazines and newspapers, as well as on radio and TV. As well as teaching Face Yoga to countless clients, I have worked with major brands around the globe. I also offer teacher-training courses and mine is the most popular and longest running Face Yoga teacher-training course worldwide.

STARTING YOUR JOURNEY

When I sat down to write this book I knew that I wanted it to be accessible and fun. I also wanted it to be based on a combination of the latest research, traditional philosophies and the experiences of real people who have tried and tested the techniques.

Everything I share with you is part of my everyday life. I use all of these techniques on myself.

A HOLISTIC LIFESTYLE

I am a great believer in the holistic approach to beauty, health and wellbeing. For truly amazing skin you need to be looking at all areas of your health, from what's going on in your mind, to what you apply to your skin, to what you eat. Make your Face Yoga a routine, a ritual and a way of expressing self-love. Make it a tool for life.

AGEING IS GOOD

Something I feel very passionate about is not being "anti ageing". I do on occasion use the term as a simple way to explain to people some of the key benefits of

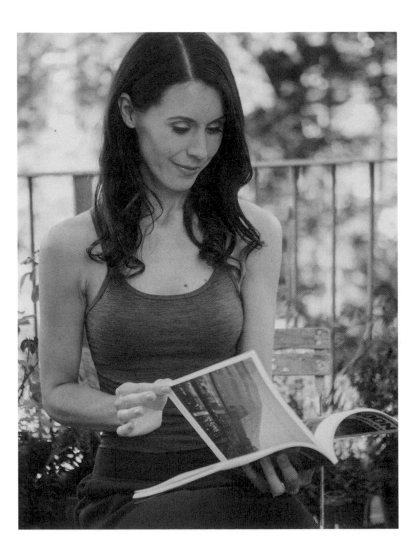

Face Yoga. But ageing itself is nothing to be ashamed of! Life is a gift and it we should be grateful for each and every day we are given. Every birthday should be celebrated with pride and joy.

DON'T HATE YOUR LINES

There isn't anything wrong with having wrinkles or lines. Every part of our face and our body changes with age. My method shows you how to prevent and reduce these things if you choose to, and if you do, please do it out of love for your face and not out of hate or fear.

A WORD ON AFFIRMATIONS

Throughout the book you will find affirmations, which are such a powerful way of moving toward a healthier, happier and calmer you. When you feel good on the inside, this radiates out through your face. Affirmations are positive statements which always start with the words "I am" and help train your mind to feel good. Don't worry if you find yourself thinking "This is not true" or "I am not that" when you repeat the affirmation. Repetition is key. Try to do at least one a day and soon they won't be just words on a page. Each affirmation should be repeated three times.

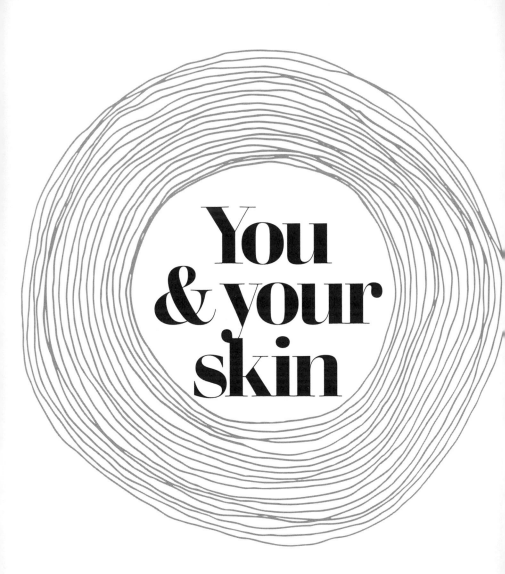

You
& your
skin

Having an understanding of your wonderful face will help you better understand why you should use Face Yoga and what changes it will make. The muscles, bones and layers of skin are a fascinating insight into the part of your body that is most recognizable: your face.

FACIAL ANATOMY

SKIN

The largest organ in the body, the skin guards us from the external elements, and protects the underlying muscles, bones and internal organs. It is made up of three layers:

1 The *epidermis*, our skin's top layer, provides a waterproof barrier that protects us from the elements and pathogens, gives us the sense of touch and regulates body temperature. It is composed of four layers of cells: the *stratum basale*, *stratum spinosum*, *stratum granulosum*, and *stratum corneum*.

2 The *dermis*, our skin's middle layer, is comprised of connective tissue which contains our collagen and elastin proteins. It also contains blood vessels, our lymphatic system, hair follicles, glands and nerves. Its main function is to protect and cushion us from stress and give our skin bounce and elasticity.

3 The *hypodermis* or bottom layer of skin is made up of connective and adipose tissue. Its main function is to protect us from trauma and cushion the skin.

In order to have healthy skin you want to give it as much help as possible to do its job. By practising Face Yoga you are helping the blood flow and the natural exfoliation of the skin through manipulation and movement. This helps the epidermis by encouraging regular shedding of the top layer. This in turn encourages the lower layer of the epidermis to produce new cells, thus helping skin to look bright, glowing and energized. Daily Face Yoga helps the *dermis* by improving the lymphatic drainage in this area which reduces puffiness, bloating and uneven skin tone.

The *hypodermis* has blood vessels and nerves like the *dermis*, so stimulation of this area helps with better circulation to the epidermis. This means vibrant skin.

MUSCLES

There are 57 muscles in the face, head and neck, including the ears and tongue. The main function of the face muscles is to give us the ability to make facial expressions.

Each muscle in the face has a particular function and needs to be looked after differently; some need to be strengthened and lifted, others need to be released of tension and some need training to stay relaxed. Face Yoga supports this amazing web of muscles in all these ways. The fact that all the muscles are attached is important, because lifting or relaxing one can provide lift and support or freedom from tension, for another.

BONES

There are 22 bones in the face and head. The function of these bones is to protect and support our face and brain. Face Yoga works less with the bones and more with the muscles and skin. However, due to the natural loss of density and thickness of some bones in the face as we age, working the muscles and skin to provide support and lift for the face is important to balance this bone atrophy and change. As the bones are attached to the muscles, strengthening and toning the muscles helps to support the bones. It has also been shown that a lack of exercise weakens bones as we age so strengthening exercises may help the bones stay strong.

WHY WE AGE

Our face ages in many ways. This section is here to give you an understanding of how internal (intrinsic) and external (extrinsic) factors can affect the skin and accelerate the ageing process.

WEATHER

Sun damage is one of the biggest causes of skin ageing. It is agreed among almost all skin experts that UV exposure can contribute to visible signs of ageing on the face. Studies have shown that even through glass and on cloudy days, UV radiation can cause skin looseness, wrinkles, lines and hyperpigmentation (sunspots).

Any extreme weather conditions can age the skin. Exposure to cold and windy environments with low humidity can dry out the skin, meaning less natural oil production and lines and wrinkles can appear more prominent. Arid, dry conditions can also mean the skin becomes dry and flaky and dead cells can accumulate on the skin.

LIFESTYLE CHOICES

SUGAR

Sorry to be the bearer of bad news but sugar is one of your skin's biggest enemies. Inflammation happens when blood sugar levels spike, which causes the skin to sag as collagen and elastin are damaged. Inflammation also aggravates spots and blemishes. Sugar permanently binds to collagen in the skin in a process called *glycation*, which causes the skin to become stiff and inflexible. This causes our face to age quicker.

If you do consume large amounts of sugar, it is key to cut down your intake to get the most out of your Face Yoga. Check labels of all foods and look for sugar or derivatives of sugar in the ingredients.

SMOKING

Smoking has devastating effects on the skin and it has been proven that a smoker's skin ages faster. There are a few reasons for this. Firstly, the repetitive movements of the pursing of the lips can cause lines around the mouth. Secondly, smoking restricts oxygen flow in the skin, starving it of nutrients and causing free radical damage. Thirdly, the chemicals present in cigarettes can destroy the collagen and elastin in the skin, making it saggier and more lined.

CAFFEINE AND ALCOHOL

Drinking alcohol, coffee, tea and other caffeinated drinks can age the skin as they are diuretics which prevent you from holding on to water. This can mean the skin becomes dry and dehydrated, and ages faster. They also increase cortisol, which can damage collagen in the skin. Caffeine and alcohol impact on our sleep too which can reduce the healing and repairing time the skin has at night. As caffeine narrows the blood vessels, the delivery of antioxidants and nutrients to the skin may be reduced. Caffeine and alcohol are mostly acidic which affects oil production in the skin, potentially contributing to acne and inflammatory skin conditions.

ANATOMY CHANGES

COLLAGEN

Collagen is the most abundant protein in the human body and is found in the connective tissue in the *dermis* (middle layer of skin) as well as in other tissues and bones. It creates flexibility and provides strength, support and structure.

Our collagen production declines with age (it is thought at around 1 per cent each year from our early twenties) and the quality also reduces. This natural decrease in production and quality is worsened by factors such as sun damage, stress, poor food choices, smoking, hormonal changes and environmental factors.

ELASTIN

Whilst collagen gives our skin firmness and strength, the protein elastin gives our skin elasticity. As we age our elastin production declines, which can leave the skin with a leathery appearance and less firmness and bounce. The skin is like a rubber band that is stretched over and over and soon loses its elasticity.

MUSCLES

The muscles in the face help give our skin lift, fullness and strength. As we age we lose muscle tone and mass. Gravity also pulls and atrophies the muscles, causing them to "fall", which results in the skin on top of the muscles becoming looser. Muscle fibres also start to shrink. Muscle tissue in the face is replaced increasingly slowly with age.

FAT

The fat in the face changes as we age. In some areas it starts to reduce and waste away, in others fat pads start to droop, and in others fat can accumulate. This causes the face to look gaunt and older in places such as the cheeks and eye sockets where we lose fat, and can mean jowls and a double chin form where fat builds.

BONE

As we age our bones show signs of shrinkage and a loss of density, which can cause our face structure to change. Bones lose calcium and other minerals, becoming weaker as a result.

CELL TURNOVER

Due to a decrease in collagen and elastin, as we age our cell turnover rate slows down. Cell turnover is the rate at which new healthy skin cells are made and the rate at which the cells in the bottom layer of skin are moved to the top layer of skin. This can result in dull, rough, dry and blemished skin.

DEHYDRATION

During ageing there is a natural dehydration of the *stratum corneum* due to a breakdown of skin cells, which causes a thinning of the *epidermis* and *dermis*. There is also a reduction in GAGs, such as hyaluronic acid (HA), in the skin. The skin makes HA to retain moisture in the cells and it has been shown to be important for hydration, nourishing collagen and lubricating of joints. Levels start to fall in our forties and due to hormonal changes there is also a natural reduction in oil production which can cause the skin to look drier and wrinkles to appear more apparent.

HORMONES

Hormones can play a part in all the changes mentioned

above. Stress hormones like cortisol and adrenaline can affect our skin, causing everything from a destruction of collagen to sluggish lymphatic drainage.

EXPRESSIONS

Expressions are linked to both verbal and non-verbal communication, thoughts and emotions as well as habits such as squinting in the sun. The repetition of these expressions over and over gradually start to form lines which become deeper as we age. Our skin's ability to "bounce back" decreases, and lines and wrinkles start to develop. One way to avoid this is to do daily Face Yoga to reduce current lines and to prevent new lines forming.

SLEEP POSITION

Sleep is essential for good skin but the wrong sleep position can cause lines on the skin. Sleeping on your side and particularly on the same side every night can cause repetitive creases and therefore lines and wrinkles on the face and neck. Try to sleep on your back or swap sides as often as you can.

SCREEN TIME

Screen time is one of the major causes of posture-related facial ageing. Bending forward to look at a phone can cause lines in the neck and when this is done multiple times a day it can age the skin.

STRESS AND NEGATIVE EMOTIONS

When we are under pressure our body goes into "fight or flight" mode, our inbuilt physical and mental response to danger of any kind. Our body reacts as though we are in a life-threatening situation. Chronic stress is exhausting for all our systems and organs and can have devastating effects on the body and mind. It can also affect the face by contributing to collagen and elastin breakdown, dehydration, stress-related expressions, muscle weakness, sluggish circulation, poor lymphatic drainage and slow cell turnover.

Negative emotions, such as sadness, grief, worry or anger, show on our face. It is hard to hide negativity that's going on inside. Along with the physical reasons how stress ages the face, the thoughts and emotions related to stress can show in many ways too.

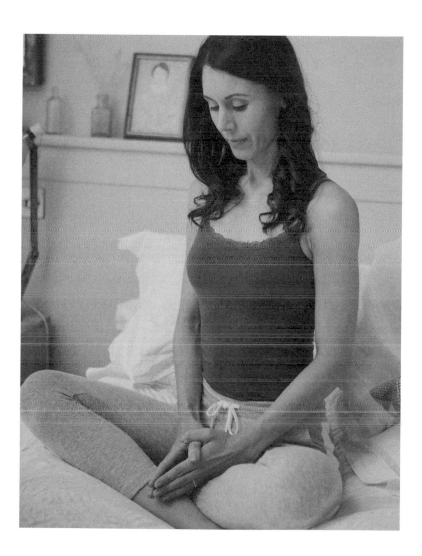

SKINCARE

Skincare is important for a healthy face and to get the best benefits from your Face Yoga. Unless you look after your skin well with a daily skincare regime, it cannot renew, repair and protect itself to the best of its ability. There are five main steps that I would highly recommend you follow for a basic skincare routine.

1. CLEANSE

Cleansing your skin every evening is vital for a healthy glow and it compliments the skin-clearing benefits of Face Yoga. Night-time cleansing helps to rid the skin of dirt, excess oil and pollution and allows it to do its vital job at night of renewing and repairing. If the grime from the day was left on the skin it could clog pores, which, once stretched to accommodate this grime, may not bounce back. Additionally, not cleansing at night can mean the skin doesn't naturally exfoliate itself, which deprives it of oxygen and causes dull skin.

When it comes to morning cleansing there are two schools of thought. Some people feel it can strip the natural oils and prefer to just splash the face with cold

For many years I suffered from very bad acne. At the age of 14 my face, neck, back and arms were covered in spots. The doctor prescribed a number of medications, one of which was such a strong topical treatment that my blue bed cover was bleached white by it! These spots plagued me to varying degrees for many years. Discovering Face Yoga in my early twenties helped me start to reduce my acne. Each year that I integrated healthier living into my life, the spots subsided just that little bit more. However, even in my early and mid thirties I noticed I was still getting two or three big spots the week before my period, which often took a whole month to shift. After lots of experimenting with what worked for me, I worked out the perfect combination of natural skincare products to compliment my Face Yoga, nutrition and wellbeing.

water. Others prefer to also cleanse in the morning, to wash away the dead skin cells and sebum that can build up during the night.

Find a cleansing routine that works for you. You can choose between oil cleansers, cream cleansers, micellar water cleansers and foam wash cleansers. Whichever product you choose, cleanse nightly (and in the morning if you want) to ensure your skin is given its best chance to renew and repair – and therefore have a gorgeous glow.

TOP TIP: choosing products that are either organic or sourced from mostly natural ingredients and never tested on animals is more beneficial for your skin, friendlier for the environment and more ethical.

2. TONE

I would highly recommend you use a toner or hydrating mist every day directly after you cleanse and just before you moisturize. If you have oily or acne-prone skin, toner can help to get rid of any remaining oil or sebum and tightens and closes the pores to reduce dirt and oil build-up which can cause spots.

If you are a makeup or sunscreen wearer, toner can remove any last traces, making sure your skin (and pores) are fully clean and therefore able to properly renew and refresh during the night. Choosing the right toner for your face is imperative. Different skin types suit different toners. For all skin types I would highly recommend an alcohol-free toner – the product should never be too astringent or harsh and the aim should be always to balance your skin's natural pH levels.

> **TOP TIP:** apply your toner or hydrating mist with organic cotton wool pads. Gently sweep over the face in an upward, outward motion.

3. MOISTURIZE

After you have cleansed and toned, the next step is to hydrate. For most skin types, an organic Soil Association accredited moisturizing serum, such as Fusion by Danielle Collins, is beneficial as it is full of proactive plant botanical oils which hydrate, smooth and support the skin's natural ability to regenerate new cells. A serum like this works well on its own but can be layered under cream moisturizer and over products like hyaluronic acid. Many serums on the market are designed to be layered with a cream moisturizer. Cream moisturizers are the most commonly used hydration products but I recommend that you look out for ones that are free from parabens, chemicals, fillers, sulphates, phthalates, silicones and alcohol. Additionally, you don't want the cream too thick otherwise it just sits on the top layer of skin.

Apply your serum and/or moisturizer using an upward motion from the décolletage all the way to the forehead. Then, with all your fingers, use a tapping action to help the product penetrate deeper into the skin.

TOP TIP: don't forget to apply product to the sides and back of your neck and make sure your product is high in antioxidants to protect from and repair free radical damage.

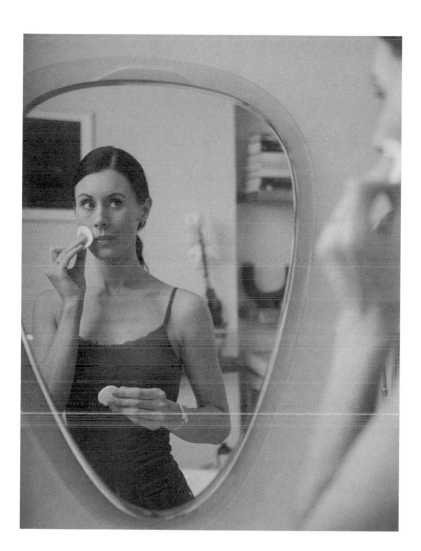

4. EXFOLIATE

Exfoliating the face regularly is essential for radiant skin. As we age the rate of cell turnover and the ability to slough of dead skin cells slows, which can result in dry, dull and rough skin and enlarged and blocked pores. As dead skin cells, makeup and dirt build up, acne and blemishes may form and wrinkles and lines may appear more prominent. Sloughing off the top layer through gentle exfoliation can help the skin appear brighter, smoother and more youthful.

How you choose to exfoliate is really down to your skin type, time and budget. You can either choose chemical exfoliation like fruit enzymes or gentle peels which absorb into the skin to regenerate cell turnover, or physical exfoliation like face scrubs which use abrasion on top of the skin. It is important not to over exfoliate; once to three times a week is ideal for most people.

TOP TIP: if you have any inflammatory skin conditions such as acne, rosacea or eczema for example, please consult a dermatologist for the best exfoliation method for you.

What works for me when it comes to sun protection and finding the balance between protecting my skin from ageing and burning and getting vitamin D is to wear SPF 30 on my face every day (on the days I wear makeup I use an SPF 20 mineral foundation on top of this). On sunny days I wear sunglasses and a hat and always wear SPF 30 on my hands. During the summer months in the UK, I expose my arms and legs for 10–20 minutes without sunscreen and then put on SPF all over or stay out of the sun. During the winter, due to the colder temperatures it makes it harder to expose my skin to the sun. Therefore I take a multivitamin with vitamin D and I also make sure that I eat vitamin D-rich foods. This is what works for me but every one is different so find what works for you.

5. SUNSCREEN

If you take away only one skincare tip from this book, make it this: always add a daily SPF for your face to your routine. This is absolutely key to preventing the harmful effects from the sun.

The SPF should be SPF 30 or over. Despite the numbers making you think differently, there is a much bigger difference between SPF 15 and SPF 30 than 30 and 50. So it doesn't matter too much whether you go for 30, 40 or 50 (just find a brand which suits).

Wear sunscreen every day, regardless of the weather. The UVA rays which age the skin can penetrate cloud and glass so even when you are driving or sat near a window, wearing sunscreen is essential.

A little note here on Vitamin D and sun exposure. Our best source of vitamin D is the sun so finding the balance between protection from both the burning and ageing rays of the sun and getting your daily dose of vitamin D is tricky. From an ageing point of view, minimum sun exposure is our best bet when it comes to keeping the skin looking young but some exposure is needed for other aspects of our health.

It is also worth remembering that you can get some vitamin D from foods and vitamin D supplements are also a way to up your intake but should of course be taken with care. Foods rich in vitamin D are oily fish, eggs, some meats and cod liver oil. If you are plant-based then mushrooms which are stored by a sunny window and vitamin D-fortified milk or milk alternatives and fortified orange juice are options.

TOP TIP: don't rely on an SPF in your serum, moisturiser or makeup. While these do provide a level of protection, they do not have the same level of protection as sunscreen. So wear SPF over your serum and moisturiser and under your makeup. Every single day.

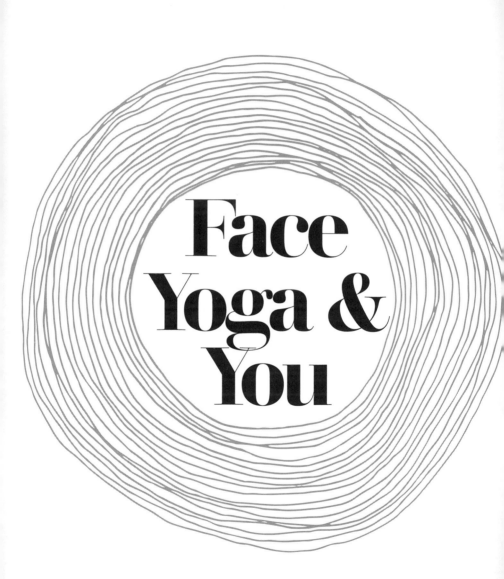

Face
Yoga &
You

How does Face Yoga work?
The five main aspects of The Danielle Collins Face Yoga Method are: face exercise, face massage, face acupressure, face relaxation and wellbeing. This section explains the importance of each.

EVIDENCE AND RESEARCH

I spent a lot of time researching and creating The Danielle Collins Face Yoga Method. I looked into techniques which had been used for thousands of years in the East – in India, China and Japan. These face exercises, face massage, acupressure and wellbeing techniques have been passed down through the generations as a way to keep the face, mind and body healthy and youthful. I also did a lot of investigation into why the face ages and what we can do about this, looking at the face muscles, the skin and the bones. Also, modern research plays a major part in my Method too. There are an emerging number of studies that have shown very positive results which I have drawn on in developing my Method. As you go through this book you will see how I fuse traditional Eastern techniques with new Western research and philosophies.

FACE EXERCISE

We all know the benefits of exercise for the body. Think of a person you know, of any age, who does regular, focused and specific strength exercises for their body. Think of how their stomach, arms, bottom or legs look. This is the simplest way of understanding how exercise can benefit a muscle.

The face exercises in The Danielle Collins Face Yoga Method also focus on relaxing and releasing tension and stress from muscles. They work on encouraging blood flow to the muscles and training the mind to consciously relax the muscles. This is important to understand because some muscles need to be strengthened and lifted and others need to be relaxed.

The muscles in the face are composed slightly differently to those in the body. They are all attached to each other, the bone or the skin and mostly controlled by the facial nerve (our body muscles on the other hand are usually controlled by our bones). This is what gives us the ability to make expressions. So our facial muscles need to be targeted slightly differently. This is why some techniques in the programme are about toning, whilst others are about relaxing. However, despite the differences in the body and face muscles, in one sense the principle is the same. If we just rely on regular day-to-day living rather than specific exercises, some muscles in our body become weak and lose tone. The same is true for the face. If we just rely on the movements from talking, facial expressing and eating, which are uncontrolled and often rooted in stress and tension, and we are not exercising or relaxing all layers of skin and muscles together as a unit, they become looser and saggier.

One of the most recent and significant studies was carried out in January 2018 by Northwestern University in the USA. Participants did 30 minutes of Face Yoga, the majority of which were facial exercises, for 20 weeks and were assessed by a team of skin and medical professionals. For those who did it daily, it showed an almost 3 year age decrease in the 20 weeks.

Face Yoga is mostly used for aesthetic and wellbeing purposes but it has started to be recommended by organizations such as the

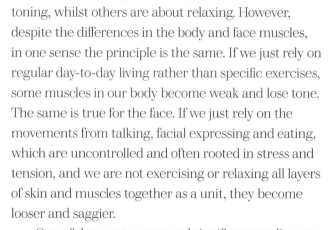

Palsy Association and the Stroke Association for rehabilitation purposes. This is because of the ability of face exercises to help the face regain strength, symmetry and improve blood flow to the skin and muscles. There was a key study done on face exercise for the elderly which concluded that facial exercises are effective in improving the mental health, facial expression and tongue muscle power of elderly people, and that exercises may be useful as a therapeutic modality in this population.

On this note, please consult a doctor if you are using Face Yoga for rehabilitation purposes.

FACE MASSAGE

Face massage plays a key role in Face Yoga. It involves using the hands to gently stimulate and manipulate the skin and muscles. It feels wonderful and gives you glowing skin

Face massage has been around since as early as the 3rd century BC and its benefits are well known, and well proven.

It may help with lymphatic drainage which means that it may help to move any stagnant lymph in the face.

This reduces under-eye bags, puffiness and bloating in the face. One study showed that this can give the skin the appearance of having had "a mini facelift" and another concluded that without manual lymphatic drainage in the face, the skin can be prone to sagging.

Face massage has been proven to increase blood flow to the skin and muscles, which has short-term benefits of a healthier and more energized appearance and the long-term benefit of better circulation.

Face massage can help the mind to feel calmer and more content. It can also reduce stress on the face, helping it look more rested and relaxed. Both these points are key in terms of anti ageing.

If you have inflammatory skin conditions such as rosacea or eczema, face massage may feel uncomfortable or even aggravate the skin. It is important to use common sense (if it doesn't feel right, don't do it) as well as seeking medical advice.

Some research has suggested that massage can increase the penetration of product into the skin, so combining a product with massage may get the most benefits out of your skincare regime.

One of the most common comments I hear from people who exercise their body regularly is, "My body and face don't match". When I ask them whether they exercise their face as frequently as they do their body, they often have a "light bulb moment". I have seen this so many times. They realize that if they are taking the time to exercise (and massage and relax) their body, they need to dedicate time to their face as well.

FACE ACUPRESSURE

Acupressure is the art of applying pressure to specific points on the face and body using the fingertips. The practice began in Asia and has formed an integral part of TCM (Traditional Chinese Medicine), Ayurveda (Indian Medicine) and Shiatsu (from Japan) for more than 5,000 years.

From an Eastern perspective, stimulating certain points can help balance our "subtle energy" or "life force energy" – something which may be tricky to measure but can certainly be felt or experienced by the individual. When the energy is flowing well we look and feel at optimum health and our body and mind are balanced and calm.

From a Western medicine perspective, the benefits of acupressure are reported to be relaxation, pain relief, muscle easing and improved blood flow. Also it is said that the placebo effect or conducting acupressure in a calming and mindful way are the reasons people look and feel better as a result. From beauty point of view, it is said that acupressure eases tension in facial muscles, which means we are less likely to frown, squint and scowl. Even if you choose to believe only these more evidence-based, pragmatic arguments, there are still plenty of reasons to do acupressure for aesthetic and wellness reasons.

The techniques in this book that are based on acupressure have been carefully selected because they are safe and have both aesthetic and wellbeing benefits. I have been using and teaching them for the past 16 years. However, if you are pregnant or have a medical condition, please consult a doctor before proceeding.

I have worked with a huge range of clients who have found the acupressure incredibly beneficial for their wellbeing and improving their skin. I hear on a weekly basis how calm clients feel after using acupressure. For this reason many people practise it before they go to sleep or in times of stress.

FACE RELAXATION

Relaxation of the face is an important aspect of Face Yoga. Tension from both physical and mental pressure can have many negative effects on both the appearance and the health of our skin.

When we are stressed, we can hold this strain in our facial muscles, causing deep-set lines and wrinkles. It is agreed amongst almost all dermatologists and doctors that expressions, when repeated over and over can in time cause lines. So relaxing is key.

There are multiple studies on the role of relaxation in reducing stress. One study showed the relaxation benefits of facial massage techniques. The study showed a significant reduction in anxiety and low mood. This is important because our facial expressions often reflect what we're feeling. Research has shown that all types of relaxation (be it mindfulness, breathing or yoga) can help relax the face but this study in particular suggested that facial massage has strong effects on stress alleviation, or psychological relaxation.

WELLBEING

The wellbeing aspects of Face Yoga are wide reaching and include nutrition, affirmations, sleep, posture, visualization, relaxation, positive thinking, yoga and skincare. An essential part of The Danielle Collins Face Yoga Method is self-care and self-love. A significant study showed that those who experience positive emotions experience higher life satisfaction. When we feel good on the inside, we look good on the outside. The final two chapters of this book are focused on this and here I draw on key studies on wellbeing.

KEY BENEFITS YOU MAY EXPERIENCE WITH FACE YOGA

1 Smoother skin
2 Firmer skin
3 Lifted muscles
4 Plumper skin
5 Reduction in lines and wrinkles
6 Reduction in puffiness and dark circles
7 Energized appearance
8 Reduction in facial tension
9 Improved skin tone
10 Less eye strain
11 Less head, neck and shoulder tension
12 Calmer mind
13 Reduction in facial, neck, shoulder and head pain
14 Better mindfulness and awareness
15 Overall feeling of wellness

USING FACE YOGA

Later in this book there are chapters focusing on specific areas of the face: the forehead, the eyes, the cheeks, the mouth, the jaw and the neck. There are also 17 dedicated solutions to common issues that Face Yoga can help with later in this chapter. Every technique in the book takes you 1 minute so here are some options how you can use them:

50 minutes: do every Face Yoga technique in the book once a day, 6-7 days a week.

30 minutes: do all 5 of the 5 chapters which work on parts of the face – forehead, eyes, cheeks, mouth, jaw and neck, 6-7 days a week.

20 minutes: do all the 17 techniques in this section, which focus on common problems, every day.

5 minutes: pick one of area of the face and work through that section. Pick a different section the following day.

1 minute: dip in to any of the techniques any time for a quick Face Yoga solution. Ideally every day.

The absolute ideal would be to do **at least** 20–30 minutes per day. A recent study showing that Face Yoga makes you look 3 years younger in 20 weeks was with participants doing 30 minutes per day. I have always recommended 20 minutes to my clients to get best results, more if needed, but remember anything is better than nothing.

FACE YOGA EVERY DAY

If I was to suggest just one thing to you it would be to **do a little every day**. Face Yoga will give you great skin but only if you actually do it and do it regularly. You can have one day to rest but if you are doing it six days a week that is perfect. Don't worry if you are instantly thinking "But how can I manage that?" I completely get where you are coming from (as a busy working mum of two girls under six!) but I promise you if you can do just 1 minute a day, you will be pleased that you have. Plus finding a little time each day, whether it is 1 minute or 50 minutes, can do wonders for your wellbeing. It gives you time and space to look after yourself, to breathe and to focus on no one else but you.

NEVER TOO EARLY OR TOO LATE

You may be wondering when is the best age to start Face Yoga. The answer is the age you are now! The benefits of starting early mean you can use it to prevent signs of ageing and have a wonderful set of techniques to use throughout life. Starting later in life is also great. It's never too late to strengthen a muscle, to improve

My oldest clients are a 92-year-old famous TV actress and a group of 91–95 year olds in a retirement village. They all enjoy finding a way to help their skin look fresher and brighter. They also like how they can do Face Yoga sitting in a chair and wearing what they like – and they have lots of fun with it too! Studies have shown that the nurturing touch of massage has beneficial wellbeing effects for the elderly.

skin tone or to boost circulation. And its always a good time to relax the mind, have a healthy body and integrate wellbeing techniques into your life.

RESULTS

Results from doing Face Yoga really do vary from person to person. There are so many factors which play a part in the speed of results, such as genes, age and lifestyle. The way that EVERYONE gets results is by doing it every day. I can't say this enough. It's the regularity of practice which plays the biggest role in seeing a smoother, firmer and healthier face.

As soon as you do your first Face Yoga session you may feel a difference: the results of the strengthening exercises on your muscles, the tension melting away and a warmth in your face from the increased blood flow to the skin.

With daily practice, you may see a notable difference in your skin within a week. Most people see some changes within a month. You may find it takes 6–8 months to see significant results. I highly recommend taking a "before" picture of yourself prior to starting the Method and then do weekly photos for a year. This is an excellent way to see the positive changes.

WILL DOING FACE YOGA HARM MY SKIN?

Face Yoga is a very safe and effective way of having healthy skin. Some people have suggested that it can give you wrinkles but this is a response to lots of unhelpful videos that are on the internet. These images show people doing what they call "Face Yoga" but who are in fact moving their face in any old direction or pulling or dragging their skin in a rough and incorrect way. My Method doesn't work in that way, for three reasons.

Firstly, you are working the muscles of the face in a slow, controlled way that ensures you are using all 3 layers of the skin and the muscles in unison with each other. You are checking that no part of the skin is creasing or wrinkling while doing it.

Secondly, you are massaging either very gently using a feather-like touch, or you are pinching down to the muscle, engaging all the layers of skin. This does not involve dragging or pulling.

Thirdly, you are training the face to relax. A big reason why we get lines is due to repeating facial expressions, over and over again. The Danielle Collins

Face Yoga Method trains you to learn how to relax your muscles and release tightness and tension – which may be causing you to pull in or raise up your eyebrows, for example. This retraining of the face is a great way to prevent lines and can even start to soften and reduce lines too.

WHEN TO DO FACE YOGA

It really doesn't matter what time of the day you do Face Yoga. If you can find a routine, a regular time each day which works for you, then you are more likely to do it every day.

People often ask me when do I do my Face Yoga. My main practice is in the evening. This works best for me, particularly since I've had children because the morning is just too rushed! I do my Face Yoga either in bed before sleep, in front of the TV or a film, or while I am in the bath.

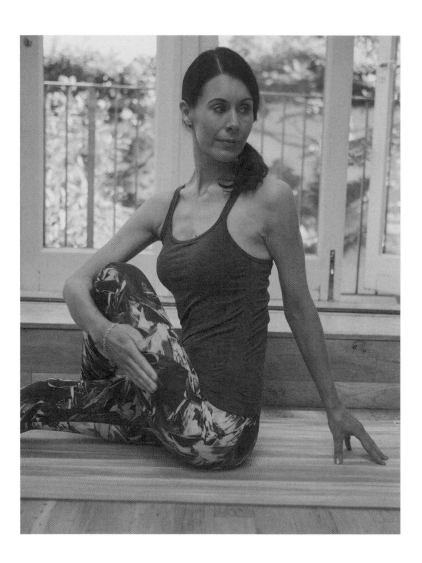

THE WORD "YOGA" IN "FACE YOGA"

So why did I choose to use the word "yoga" in The Danielle Collins Face Yoga Method, rather than call it "Face Exercise" for example?

Yoga means "union" and my Method is very much a union of techniques. It also has strong wellbeing, self-care and holistic lifestyle elements to it which are all an important part of yoga.

Some of my first training was as a yoga teacher and this had a strong influence on The Danielle Collins Face Yoga Method.

Face Yoga is in fact rooted in traditional yoga practice but it wasn't brought across to the West in the 1960s and 1970s with the more physical body movements. Many aspects of the Method derive from Eastern philosophies and therapies. It has a modern twist but incorporates the breath, mediation, concentration, positivity, posture and a state of being in the moment that are all part of traditional yoga.

SAFETY

The first point I would make when it comes to safety is listen to your face, body and mind. If you ever feel any discomfort or pain, or your gut instinct says something isn't right for you, always listen to that. It is fine to stop and rest, skip a technique or do fewer repetitions. If you have any medical conditions or skin problems, please always check with a doctor prior to starting Face Yoga. Face Yoga is simple, gentle and effective but you are unique so learn what is best for you. You shouldn't hold tension in any part of the face other than the 'workout' feeling you will get when strongly exercising a certain muscle. Constantly scan your face for tension and consciously release any you find. Also always use a mirror, you shouldn't be creating any expression lines while doing Face Yoga. If you notice any, adjust the exercise, ease off a little or use your fingers to smooth that area.

YOUR TOP FACE YOGA TIPS

1 Always wash your hands before starting to prevent the spread of bacteria.

2 Remove all makeup and apply a small amount of a plant-based moisturizing serum. Apply slightly less than usual so your fingers don't slip.

3 Take weekly side and front-on pictures of yourself and you will be able to track any changes.

4 If it feels more comfortable for you, remove glasses or contact lenses.

5 Use a mirror to check for any tension or expression lines and consciously smooth these out.

6 Have good posture throughout.

7 Have fun with the techniques. It's not a problem if you laugh!

8 Breathe deeply in through the nose, letting the abdomen rise and out through the nose, letting the abdomen fall. Make the exhalation longer than the inhalation.

9 Follow a healthy lifestyle to get the best results.

10 Get to know your face and learn to relax it so you don't create expression lines in your daily life.

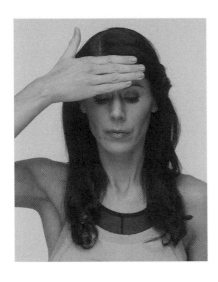

THE FOREHEAD DAB

- - - -

1 Start with your eyes either open or closed – whichever feels more comfortable.

2 Place the palm of your hand on the right side of your forehead. Press, or "dab", your forehead gently, moving gradually across to the left, then back toward the right.

3 Start with one dab per second, then gradually slow it down to one dab every 10 seconds. Do this exercise for 1 minute in total.

✳ BENEFITS

Relaxing the frontalis muscle of your forehead means less tension. This exercise also improves circulation, keeping the skin refreshed and glowing.

✳ TOP TIP

Use this exercise to practise keeping your forehead still while widening the eyes – a great way to avoid expression lines.

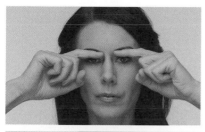

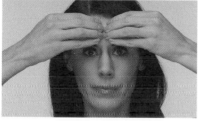

THE
EYEBROW
LIFT

- - - -

1 Place your two index fingers under the eyebrows. Very slowly close your eyes and hold for 10 seconds. Repeat twice more. You should feel a shaking in the upper part of your eyelids.

2 Lift your hands away from the eyebrows and place all your finger tips in the middle of the forehead. Very gently smooth the fingers away from each other toward your temples and then lift off. Keep the eyes wide and don't raise the eyebrows. Repeat for 30 seconds.

✳ BENEFITS

The muscles in your forehead work against the resistance of the finger which helps to build strength and tone.

✳ TOP TIP

Because this exercise asks you to raise your eyebrows it should be followed by a forehead massage to ensure that the forehead muscle is relaxed following the exercise.

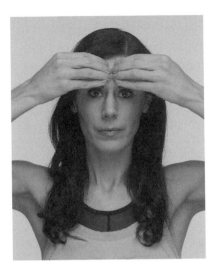

THE
BUTTERFLY

----

1 Using your index finger, middle finger and ring finger on both hands, smooth the forehead. Move your hands away from each other and when they reach the hair line, look down and hold for 10 seconds.

2 Bring the fingers back to your starting position and repeat twice more.

3 Now do the same exercise (3 sets of 10 seconds) but with your eyes wide open, ensuring you don't raise the eyebrows.

✳ BENEFITS

The massaging action helps to relieve tension in your procerus muscle which runs between your eyebrows, which can prevent lines being formed.

✳ TOP TIP

Try not to drag the skin too much with this exercise.

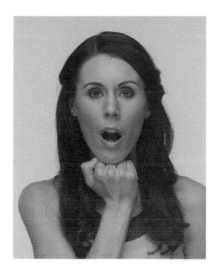

BENEFITS

This exercise works on toning and strengthening many of your lower face muscles and the fist acts as resistance to work the muscles in the lower jaw area.

TOP TIP

If it feels more comfortable you can rest your elbow on a table.

THE THINKER

- - - -

1 Make a fist and place it under your chin, pushing upward slightly.

2 Open and close your mouth 30 times. Keep pushing upward with your hand slightly. Your chin should be parallel to the floor.

3 Now hold your mouth open, and very slightly wrap your lips around your teeth. Hold for 30 seconds.

I AM
peaceful

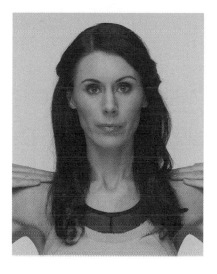

EASE THE SHOULDERS

- - - -

1 Place your hands on your shoulders and start to roll the shoulders back, slowly 15 times, only rolling as far as is comfortable for you.

2 Then roll your shoulders forward 15 times.

✳ BENEFITS

This exercise helps to ease tightness and muscle strain in your shoulders, which can reduce and prevent tension. It may also help to improve posture and reduce and prevent neck tension.

✳ TOP TIP

Do this exercise especially when at a computer and before tension builds up.

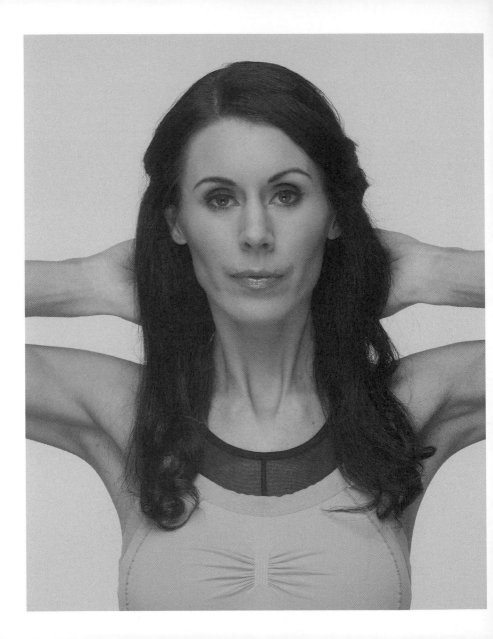

PRESS THE NECK

- - - -

1 Place your four fingers of both hands behind the back of the neck, gently pressing in to the muscles either side of your spine and tilt your head back so that the fingers press in to the muscles a little deeper. Bring your head back to the starting position and repeat again, slowly and with control. Do this 30 times in total.

2 Then hold your hands in position and tilt your head back and hold there, wiggling the fingers a bit, perhaps even doing some little circular massages. Do whatever feels intuitively right to release your neck.

✳ BENEFITS

Massaging the muscles in your neck can relieve tension, stress and even pain. This can help your neck to feel more comfortable in the short term but can also prevent tension in the long term – not only in your neck but also in your jaw and cheeks.

✳ TOP TIP

If your arms ache, relax them for a while and lift them up again when ready.

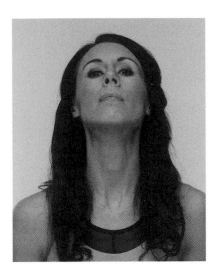

**FOR PREVENTING AND
REDUCING A TURKEY NECK**

TURKEY
NECK
TONER

----

1 Tilt your head back as far as is comfortable for you. Gently close your lips. Repeatedly bring the tip of your tongue up to the roof of your mouth and back down. Do this 60 times for 1 minute.

* **BENEFITS**

The repeated movement of the tongue engages the area under your chin, tighening loose skin as it is exercised.

* **TOP TIP**

This is quite a strong exercise so start with 30 seconds and build up when you feel ready.

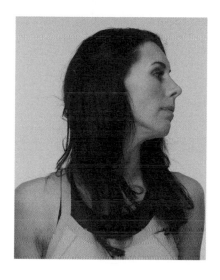

THE BIRD

- - - -

1 Turn your head and then
slightly tilt it back. Repeatedly
bring the tip of your tongue up to
the roof of your mouth and back
down for 30 seconds.

2 Come back to centre and
repeat on the other side.

✳ BENEFITS

The combination of the tongue
movement combined with
the turn and tilt of the neck
strengthens your neck and jaw
muscles to firm and tighten
loose skin in this area.

✳ TOP TIP

Make sure your chin points up
to the ceiling slightly during
this exercise.

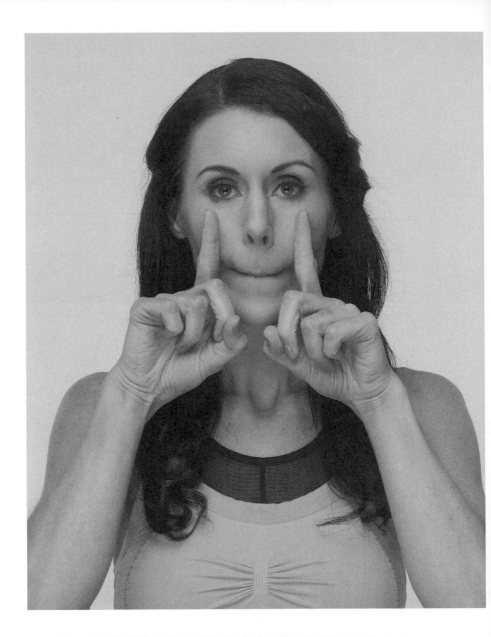

THE LIP TUCK

- - - -

1 Tuck your lips inwards (so if you looked in a mirror you wouldn't see them). Slightly lift up your lips corners, ensuring you are doing this equally both sides.

2 Use your index fingers to smooth the skin to the side of the mouth and under the mouth. Hold for 1 minute or less if it feels a lot at first.

✳ BENEFITS

This exercise strengthens the muscles in your cheeks on both sides of the face and lifts and tones the mouth muscles. It helps the face get used to using both sides equally, which helps readdress any imbalances that can build up in daily life.

✳ TOP TIP

A mirror really helps with this technique to ensure you are curling the corners of the lips up equally and that you are smoothing the skin on the lower face enough.

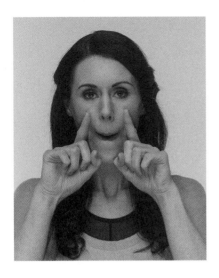

CHEEK AND JAW LIFT

----

1 Wrap your lips around your teeth and make a smile shape, lifting the corners of your lips upward so you feel this working in your cheeks.

2 Use your index fingers to smooth the skin around your cheeks and create some resistance. Hold for 30 seconds, relax and repeat once more, doing 1 minute in total.

✳ BENEFITS

This strengthens, lifts and tones the muscles around your cheek and jaw area.

✳ TOP TIP

Even if you haven't got sallow cheeks, this is a lovely technique for lifting the cheek and jaw area.

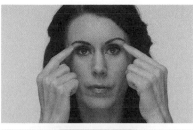

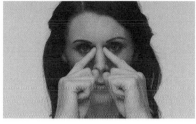

EYE DE-PUFFER

- - - -

1 Place your index fingers just under the outer edge of the eyebrows, then very gently smooth the fingers under your eyes and pause at the the inner corners for 10 seconds, pressing this acupressure point.

2 Continue in a circle down under your eye and back to this acupressure point again, pausing for 10 seconds here each time. Keep the massage going for 1 minute.

✳ BENEFITS

This helps to promote lymphatic drainage around your eye area and reduce puffiness and water retention.

✳ TOP TIP

A light touch here is key. Make sure you don't drag the skin at all. Doing it gently will be more effective for lymphatic drainage and prevent harm to your delicate eye area.

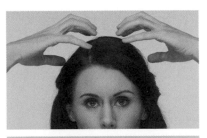

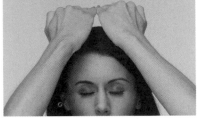

FLUFFY HEAD

----

1 Place the tips of all your fingers and both your thumbs on your head. Press and squeeze and then lift the fingers off in a flicking motion. Move to different places on the head and repeat for 30 seconds in total.

2 Then place the palms of your hands on your head and just relax them there. Close your eyes and breathe deeply in and out through your nose. Visualize tension melting away.

✳ BENEFITS

This helps to ease tension in your head and promotes feelings of relaxation through nurturing touch and breath.

✳ TOP TIP

Be intuitive with the massage. If you feel the need to go deeper or massage in a circular motion then this is fine.

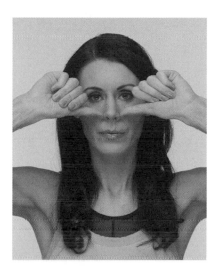

THE SINUS RELEASE

- - - -

1 Place your thumbs on the acupressure point either side of the nostrils – you will feel a slight indentation there. Hold for 30 seconds.

2 Slide your thumbs upward and outward, stopping before you get to the skin around the delicate eye area. Lift your thumbs off, then place them back at the starting position and continue this massage for 30 seconds in total.

✳ BENEFITS

This stimulates an acupressure point renowned for helping with sinus issues, relieving tension and pain, and helping to release blocked mucous. It also promotes vibrant and glowing cheeks.

✳ TOP TIP

Take a few deep breaths through your nose afterwards to further clear your sinuses.

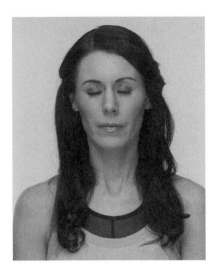

THE BREATH RETENTION

- - - -

1 Inhale through your nose and let your abdomen rise. Pause for a couple of seconds. Exhale through your nose, making the out breath longer than the in breath. Pause for a couple of seconds.

2 Repeat this sequence for 1 minute, only retaining the breath for as long as is comfortable for you.

✳ BENEFITS

This yogic breath helps to slow down your breathing, making you feel calmer. The benefits of this type of deep breathing have been proven by multiple studies to relieve stress and anxiety, and to boost the mood.

✳ TOP TIP

Ensure your face is fully relaxed throughout the technique.

I AM
happy

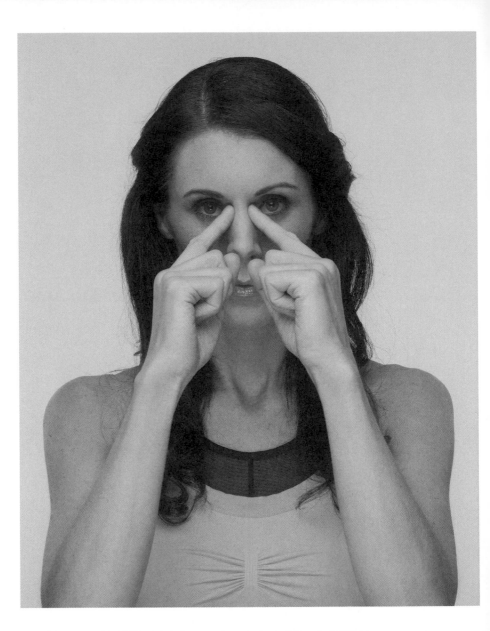

INNER EYE ACUPRESSURE

- - - -

1 Place your index fingers at the inner corners of your eyes, on the edge of the upper nose where there is a natural indentation. Press gently here, breathing deeply and hold for 30 seconds.

2 Then massage in one direction for 15 seconds and then the other direction for 15 seconds, making sure the circles are very small.

✷ BENEFITS

Acupressure has been used for thousands of years and is proven to helps reduce stress and anxiety and improve sleep. The inner-eye area can hold a lot of tension so it feels very calming to press and massage here. Combined with deep breathing in and out through the nose this is a wonderful technique to use before bed.

✷ TOP TIP

This technique is also great to reduce eye strain and helps ease headache tension.

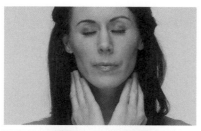

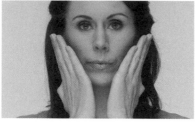

THE HANDY FACE LIFT

- - - -

1 Start by holding your hands on your neck for 20 seconds. Let the warmth of the hands relax the neck muscles and breathe deeply in and out through the nose, visualizing fatigue melting away.

2 Then, using your fingers and palms, start stroking the cheeks upward, without dragging the skin, for 20 seconds.

3 Then do the same with the forehead, stroking upward with the hands for 20 seconds.

✳ BENEFITS

This technique helps you to feel more energized and awake. It also promotes better circulation in the face, helping the skin look less tired.

✳ TOP TIP

This technique works really well when you have just applied a mositurizer, serum or oil because it helps the product sink in to the skin.

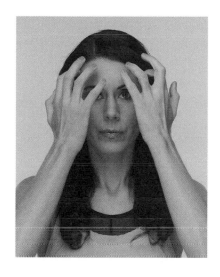

BENEFITS

This technique can instantly make your face look more vibrant and healthy due to the increased blood flow to the top layer of skin. It also releases tension build-up in your muscles.

TOP TIP

Do this first thing in the morning to start the day with a healthy glow.

FOR REDUCING AND
PREVENTING DULL SKIN

TAPPING
OVER FACE

- - - -

1 Using the tips of all your fingers start tapping over your forehead for 20 seconds.

2 Next, tap over your cheeks, mouth and jaw area for 20 seconds.

3 Finally tap all over your neck for 20 seconds.

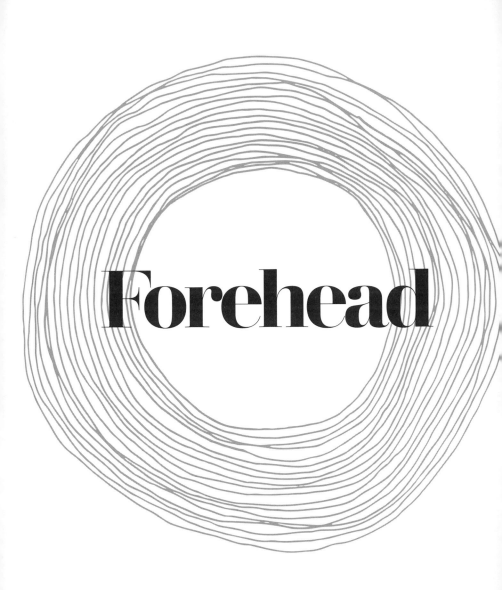

Forehead

One of the major reasons we get deep-set lines and wrinkles in the forehead area is our facial expressions. Raising the eyebrows and furrowing the brow on a daily, even hourly, basis means that the skin starts to crease and wrinkle. As we age and have less collagen and elastin, our skin's ability to bounce back from expressions decreases. But daily Face Yoga for the forehead area is a great way to help with this problem. Awareness and relaxation are key ways to prevent forehead lines. If there are already lines in this area or you want to work at preventing them, the following techniques will help.

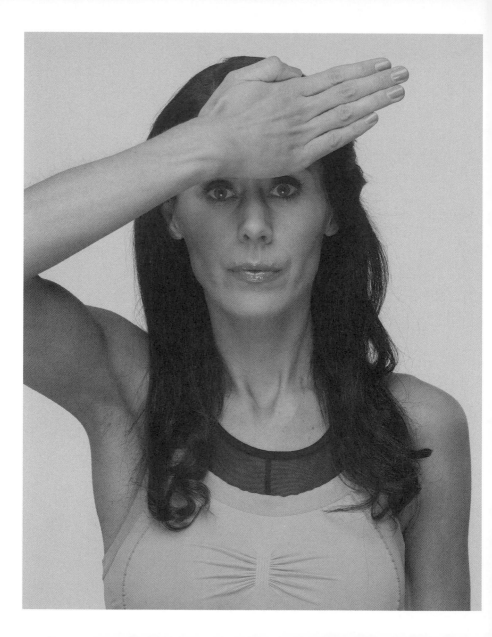

THE PALM STROKE

----

1 Start by making sure your forehead is completely relaxed and you are not lifting your eyebrows. Your eyes can be open or closed, whichever you prefer.

2 Place the palm of your hand on the middle of the forehead and slide it across. Then lift it off and use the palm of your other hand and slide this hand the other way.

3 Keep this going for 1 minute by alternating hands for each stroke, being careful not to drag your skin too much.

✳ BENEFITS

This massage is excellent for relaxing tension in the frontalis muscle in your forehead. By relaxing this muscle you are less likely to create expression lines in the area, or get tension-related headaches. The massaging action is also excellent for improving circulation, which helps to brighten your skin.

✳ TOP TIP

Take a moment to notice how your forehead muscles feel when they are completely relaxed. Then, at certain points in your day, check whether you are still maintaining this relaxation. If not, take a minute to do The Palm Stroke.

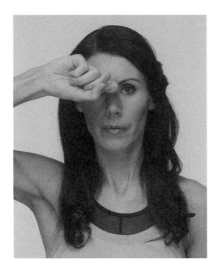

FROWN LINE SMOOTHER

----

1 Make your index fingers into little hook shapes. Then, using your knuckles, stroke upward along your procerus muscle between your eyebrows. Start from the little dip at the top of the nose and stroke all the way up to your hairline at the top of the forehead. Keep doing this massage motion, only moving in an upward direction, for 1 minute.

✳ TOP TIP

Be intuitive with the pressure you use here. You don't want to press so hard that you drag the skin too much but you don't need to keep it too soft. Find a pressure somewhere in between which feels comfortable yet energizing.

✳ BENEFITS

Massaging this area helps to encourage the muscle between your eyebrows to relax, meaning you are less likely to furrow the brow and therefore reducing lines. It also helps to smooth any existing lines and brighten your skin by improving the flow of fresh blood, nutrients and oxygen to the area.

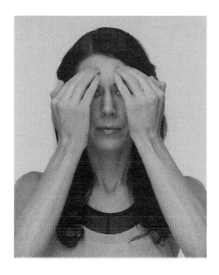

THE FOREHEAD WALK

----

1 Evenly space the index, middle and ring finger of both hands on your eyebrows. Press and take a deep breath, in and out through your nose. Move up your forehead, 1 cm at a time to the hairline, taking a deep breath, lasting 10 seconds, with each press. Repeat a second time. This exercise should last around 1 minute.

✳ BENEFITS

This technique helps to brighten your forehead area and balance your mind. It presses on lots of acupressure points which has been shown to reduce stress, insomnia and tension headaches. The gentle pressure also helps to relax tense muscles, reducing expression lines.

✳ TOP TIP

After the exercise you may see a little redness in your forehead. This is because you have improved blood flow to the top layer of skin. Never press too hard though, gentle pressure is sufficient to see good results.

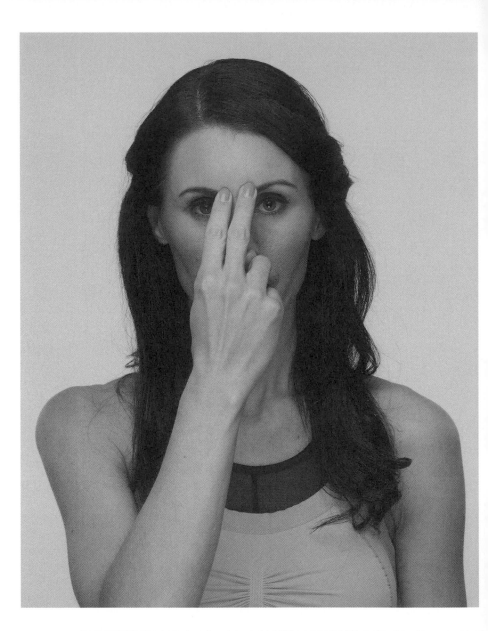

THE FROWN PREVENTER

----

1 Place your middle finger and index finger between your eyebrows. Press the fingers down to the muscle and slightly move the fingers away from each other. Hold for 20 seconds.

2 Release the fingers and repeat twice more, doing 1 minute in total.

✱ BENEFITS

This exercise is a wonderful way to reduce and prevent vertical lines between your eyebrows. It stimulates the muscle, increasing circulation to the area. It also relaxes muscle tension, which is excellent for preventing lines.

As you massage this area, you are massaging a few acupressure points which are renowned in Eastern medicine for calming the mind.

✱ TOP TIP

This is such a soothing and relaxing exercise. To further reap the calming effects, close your eyes and breathe deeply in and out through the nose throughout.

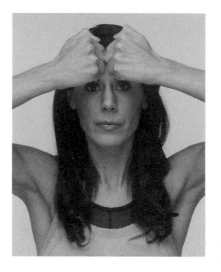

THE FOREHEAD SMOOTHER

----

1 Make both your hands into fists. Place them in the middle of the forehead. Move them outwards, away from each other, with gentle pressure. Lift them off the forehead and back to the starting position. Continue for 1 minute.

* BENEFITS

This exercise helps to ease tension in the forehead area, reducing muscle tightness.

* TOP TIP

As you do this, try widening your eyes to strengthen your eye muscles and use it as a practice to open the eyes without raising the eyebrows.

I AM
strong

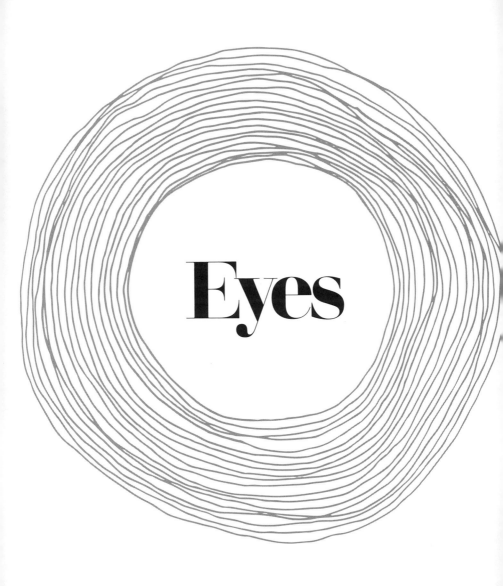

Eyes

The skin around the eyes, also known as the periocular area, is 10 times thinner than the skin on the rest the face. It's therefore much more delicate and more likely to show signs of ageing. Lines can be created from expressions such as smiling and squinting; the breakdown of collagen and elastin due to internal and external influences; and rubbing the area, for example when removing makeup or contact lenses, or with allergies. Vigorous rubbing causes tiny tears in the capillaries, leading to discoloration and puffiness.

The eye area is prone to puffiness and dark circles as well as hooded eyebrows and sunken eyes. The skin can look dehydrated and show lines earlier than other parts of the face, partially due to less oil glands. The five following exercises can help with many of these issues.

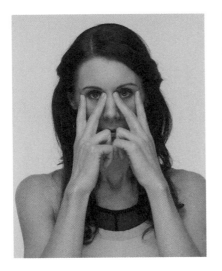

THE MINI "V"

----

1 Place your two middle fingers in the natural indentation by the inner corner of the eye at the edge of the nose. With gentle pressure, slightly bend the index fingers, and place them on the outer corner of your eye.

2 Now, look upward and make a strong squint, as though you are moving the lower eyelids upward. You should feel a little "pulse" or "shake" at the outer edge of your eye. Hold for 3 seconds and release. Continue for 1 minute, doing less if that suits you.

✳ BENEFITS

This strengthens your orbicularis oculi muscle and increases blood flow, helping your eye area appear smoother.

✳ TOP TIP

As you do the exercise, try not to pull in the area between the eyebrows or raise the eyebrows. If you don't feel the pulse at first, don't worry, in time you will do.

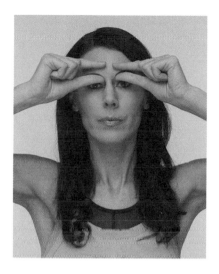

THE EYEBROW LIFTER

----

1 Using your index finger and thumb, pinch the inner edge of your eyebrows, aiming to feel right down to the muscle under the skin. Hold for 3 seconds and move along the eyebrows to the outer edge.

2 Now lift your fingers off the eyebrows and come back to the starting position, repeating again. Continue for 1 minute. If you find it more relaxing, you can close your eyes throughout.

✳ BENEFITS

This helps to reduce tension in your eyebrow area, reducing the likelihood of stress-related expression lines between the eyebrows. It also has a temporary and, with regular practice, a more long-term lifting effect of the muscle.

✳ TOP TIP

As you do this, be careful not to raise the eyebrows.

EYE SHAPES

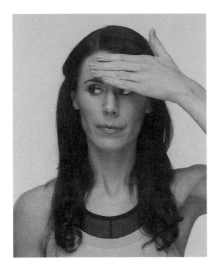

1 Place one hand on your forehead, using as much pressure as you need to stop yourself raising the eyebrows. Then move your eyes around in a circle, going clockwise and then anti clockwise. The only part of your face which is moving is the eyes.

2 Next, do the same thing with a diamond shape. Start by looking upward, then move your eyes to the right, then downwards, then to the left and then back to the top. Repeat the other way.

3 Finally, open your eyes as wide as you can, without raising the eyebrows, for 10 seconds. Repeat the circle, diamond and eyes wide position one more time both ways. The full exercise takes 1 minute.

✳ **BENEFITS**
This trains the eyes to move without moving the forehead. Practise this to reduce repetitive expressions which cause lines. It also strengthens your orbicularis oculi muscle, lifting the eye area.

✳ **TOP TIP**
This is great to do when your eyes feel tired or you have been using screens a lot.

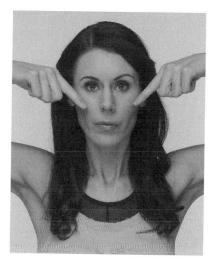

GO CROW

----

1 Start by placing the side of your index fingers on the upper part of your cheeks. With a feather-like touch, slide your fingers upward in a diagonal line until the tips are at the hairline. Continue for 30 seconds.

2 Go back to your starting position and hold there for 30 seconds, pressing gently.

✳ BENEFITS

This light massage helps to gently exfoliate the upper layer of your epidermis, increasing cell turnover. This potentially increases the thickness of this very thin skin. It also relieves tension, reducing the chance of stress-related expression lines.

✳ TOP TIP

Use a plant-based oil or eye gel to help the fingers glide.

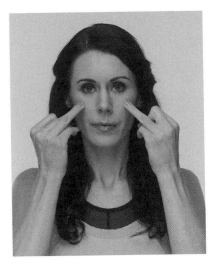

EYE DETOX MASSAGE

----

1 Using your ring finger, start gently tapping under the eye, moving inwards towards the inner corner of the eye.

2 Keep tapping, moving under your eyebrow and towards the outer edge of your eye and then move back round under your eye. Keep going with these light quick taps in this direction for 1 minute.

✳ BENEFITS

This helps with lymphatic drainage and improves blood flow, which may help to reduce and prevent dark circles and puffiness under your eye area.

✳ TOP TIP

Great to do when you first wake up to help reduce any puffiness that has built up during the night.

I AM
loved

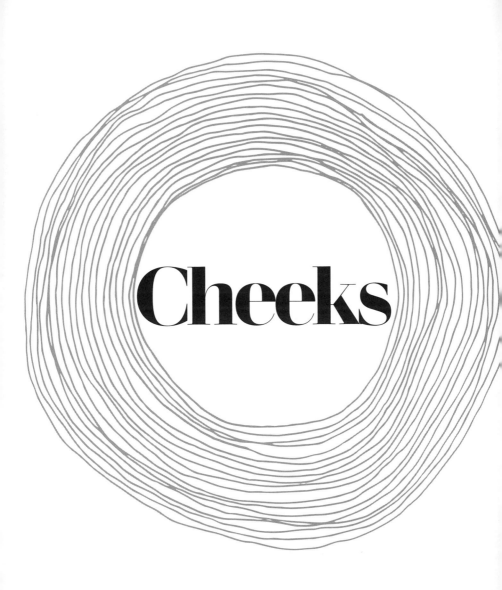

Cheeks

Taking some time each day to work on the cheek area is an important part of your Face Yoga routine. As we age, fat pads in the cheeks tend to descend and atrophy, causing the face to look gaunt and the nasal labial folds, the lines that extend from the outer corners of the nose down to the outer corners of the mouth, to deepen. Fat and bone changes can even negatively affect the area under the eyes and around the jaw. Although we can't stop these changes completely, we can strengthen and lift the muscles underneath the fat, which gives a lifted, youthful appearance and acts as "stuffing" under the skin. Two techniques in this chapter work on strengthening and lifting the muscles and the three massage techniques are great for helping the skin to look more energized and glowing.

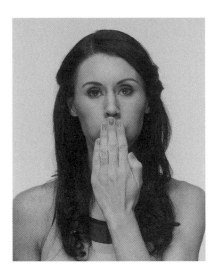

HAMSTER CHEEKS ADVANCED

----

1 Puff your cheeks out full of air. Use your fingers on one hand to ensure the skin around the lip area stays taut. Use a mirror to check you aren't crinkling the mouth area. Transfer the air from cheek to cheek, while breathing in and out through the nose. Do this for 30 seconds, then take a break for a few seconds and repeat again for 30 seconds. Work up to doing this exercise for a full minute, without stopping halfway through.

* BENEFITS

Regular practice helps to strengthen the cheek area. The fingers on your lips acts as resistance, encouraging the muscles to work harder.

* TOP TIP

If you are new to working the face muscles, you may find you need to stop a few times during the exercise. If you do, don't worry – just keep going.

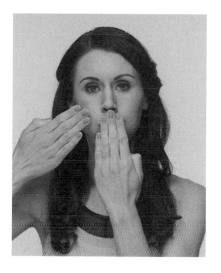

PUFFER FISH ADVANCED

----

1 Puff your cheeks out full of air. Use the fingers on one hand to ensure the skin around the lip area stays taut. Use a mirror to check you aren't crinkling the mouth area. Hold the air equally in both cheeks and use your other hand to tap one cheek for 30 seconds and then your other cheek for 30 seconds.

✳ BENEFITS

This is both a strengthening exercise to lift and firm your cheeks and an invigorating face massage to improve the circulation in the cheek area.

✳ TOP TIP

Aim to tap as much of your cheek area as possible, rather than staying in just one place. Use gentle pressure throughout.

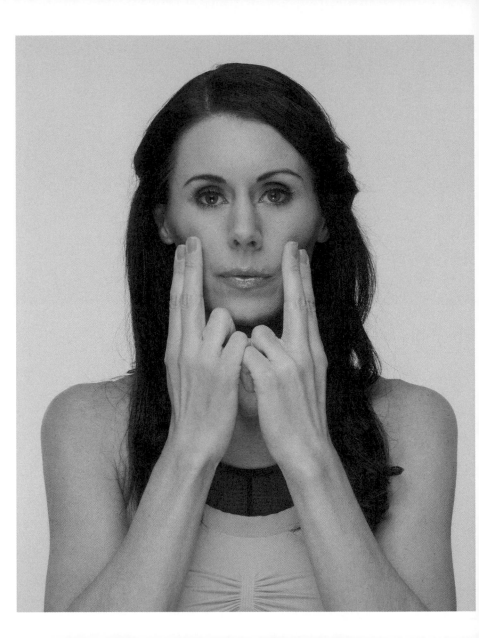

THE CHEEKBONE FLICK

----

1 Place your index and middle fingers underneath your cheekbones by the side of your nose. Press in and under your cheekbones slightly for 3 seconds. Then using a flicking motion, flick the fingers off, move across and repeat again.

2 Work up the cheeks, following the line of the cheekbone. When you can't go any further, repeat, moving upward only. Continue for 1 minute.

✳ BENEFITS

After doing this exercise you can see and feel a wonderful warmth in your cheeks, so it can help the skin look vibrant and glowing.

✳ TOP TIP

Do this whenever your skin is looking tired or dull for an instant energizing boost. It works particularly well in the morning.

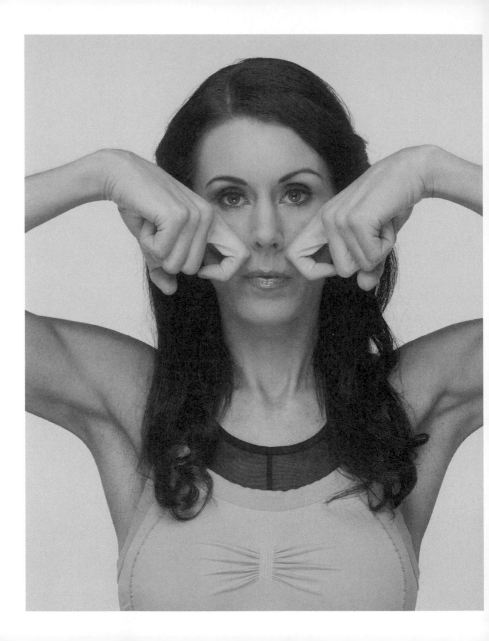

THE CHEEKBONE HOOK

----

1 Make your index fingers into hooks. Place the knuckle of each index finger underneath the cheekbones by the side of the nose. Press in and under your cheekbones and gently slide the knuckle upward and outward, following the line of the cheekbones. When you get to the end of each cheekbone, repeat again, moving upward only. Continue for 1 minute.

✳ **BENEFITS**

This exercise is excellent for releasing tension in the muscles in your cheeks. It also helps your cheeks to look brighter and more energized.

✳ **TOP TIP**

Use a plant-based oil to help the fingers glide more smoothly.

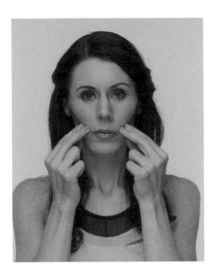

NASAL LABIAL PINCH

----

1 Using your index finger, middle finger and thumb of each hand, pinch the area either side of mouth at the corners of your lips.

2 Move upward, along the lines between your mouth and your nose to the area on the outer edge of the nostrils. Go back to the starting position and repeat, moving upward. Continue for 30 seconds. Then move the fingers 1 cm (½ inch) away from the mouth. Repeat the same thing, for 30 seconds.

✳ BENEFITS

This pinching action is great to help plump and firm the skin around the nasal labial folds.

✳ TOP TIP

Make sure you pinch down to the muscle, rather than pinching the skin outwards.

I AM
glowing

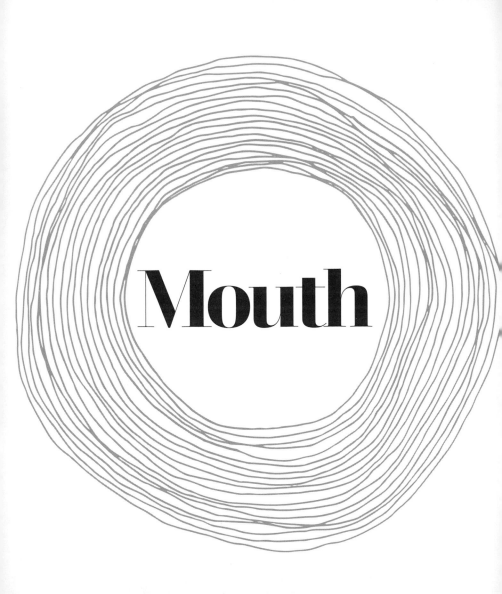

Mouth

The mouth area shows signs of aging in three main ways. Firstly, the little vertical lines around the lips sometimes known as "smoker lines". Secondly, the lips can become thinner as we age. Again this is partly due to less collagen production, as well as a reduction in hyaluronic acid and general moisture levels. Thirdly, the nasal labial folds (between the nose and mouth) and marionette lines (between the mouth and jaw) start to deepen.

In this chapter you have the Tongue Twister and the Mouth Diamond which help to strengthen the muscles around the mouth, supporting and lifting the skin. The Raindrop exercise is great for smoothing nasal labial and marionette lines and the Lip Line Circles and the Lip Plumper massage techniques help to smooth mouth lines and maintain firmness and plumpness in the lips.

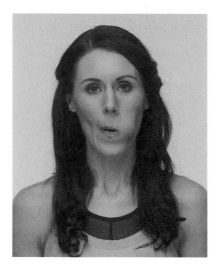

THE TONGUE TWISTER

----

1 Press your tongue into one of the corners of your mouth. Move your tongue around the lip area in a circle, very slowly, pushing the tongue toward the lips as much as possible.

2 Move in the opposite direction. Keep this going for 30 seconds. Then completely relax your mouth area. Allow every muscle to feel completely free from tension whilst breathing deeply in and out through the nose.

✳ BENEFITS

This exercise works by strengthening and toning the orbicularis oris muscle which runs around the mouth.

✳ TOP TIP

The slower you go, the more you will feel this technique working. Don't worry if your tongue aches whilst doing it, this is normal!

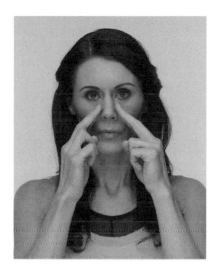

THE RAINDROP

----

1 With your mouth closed and relaxed, place your index fingers on the edge of the nose, as shown in the picture. Gently smooth the fingers down and around the edge of your mouth until the fingers meets under the mouth, imagining you are drawing a raindrop shape. Then, using slightly more pressure, massage back upward, following the same line. Continue for 30 seconds. Now, make your mouth into an "O" shape, wrapping the lips around your teeth. Do the same massage motion for 30 seconds.

✳ BENEFITS

This helps to reduce smile lines between your nose and mouth and helps to strengthen the muscle around the mouth.

✳ TOP TIP

Use gentler pressure on the way down and deeper pressure on the way up.

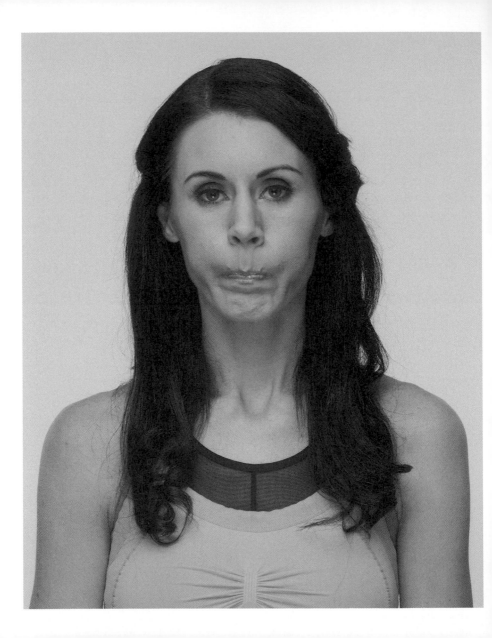

THE MOUTH DIAMOND

- - - -

1 After applying lip balm, close your mouth and puff air up into the area above the top lip. Hold for 3 seconds, breathing in and out through the nose.

2 Move the air to one cheek and hold for 3 seconds. Next, puff out the area under the lips. Lastly, move the air to the other cheek. Come back to the top again and do the same thing but in the other direction. Continue this sequence for 1 minute.

✳ BENEFITS

This helps to strengthen the muscles around the cheek and mouth area, which has a lifting and firming effect.

✳ TOP TIP

If you notice any little lines around your lips whilst doing the exercise, use your fingers on one hand to tauten the skin.

LIP LINE CIRCLES

----

1 Apply your lip balm. Using your index finger, massage the edge of your lips in a circular motion. After you have done about three circles in one spot, glide the finger across a little bit and keep going all around the lip edge. When you arrive back at your starting position, repeat in the other direction. Continue this sequence for 1 minute and apply lip balm again afterward.

✱ BENEFITS

This improves the blood flow around your lips, helping your lips appear smoother and fuller. It may also reduce lip lines.

✱ TOP TIP

After the exercise, try exfoliating your lips before applying lip balm. Use either a shop-bought exfoliator or a little olive oil and sugar mixed together.

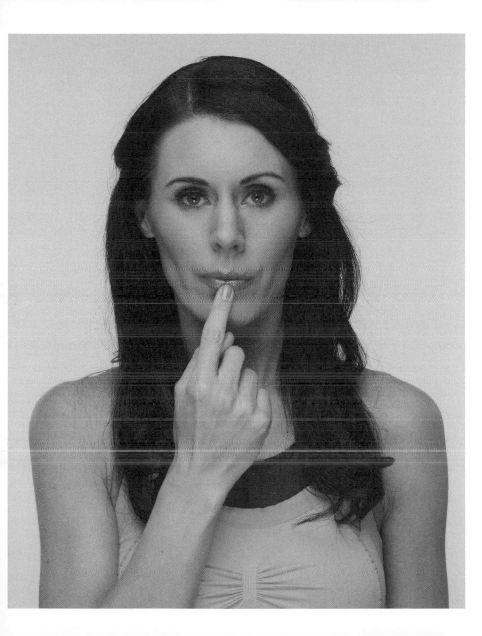

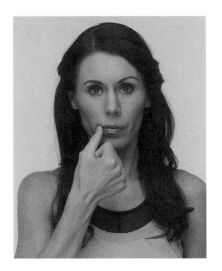

THE LIP PLUMPER

- - - -

1 Apply your lip balm. Place your thumb on the area where your lip meets your skin. Using a flicking motion, move the thumb all the way around your lips.

2 Now repeat in the other direction. You will be using downward flicks on the bottom lip and upward flicks on the top lip. Continue this sequence for 1 minute and apply lip balm again.

✱ BENEFITS
This helps to bring fresh blood and oxygen to the skin and muscle around the lip area.

✱ TOP TIP
Try not to lick your lips during your daily life. Digestive enzymes in the saliva quickly dehydrate the lips.

I AM
BEAUTIFUL
INSIDE
AND
OUT

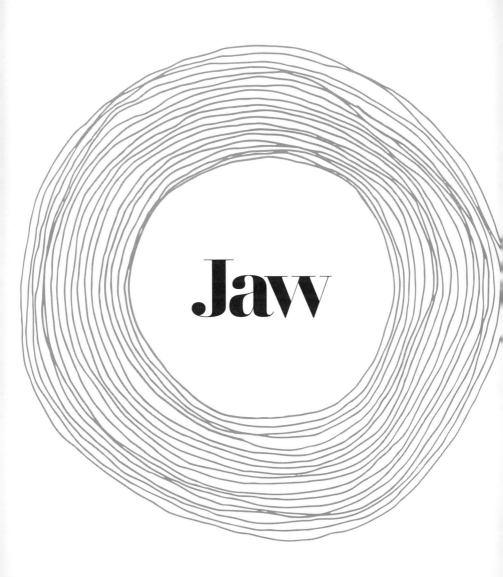

Jaw

The jaw area often holds stress and tension. Without realizing it we can clench our jaw and tighten our mouth, which can cause a tight, uncomfortable masseter muscle (one of the muscles involved in chewing), teeth grinding, TMJ disorders (which can cause pain in your jaw joint and in the muscles that control jaw movement) and headaches. The skin around the jaw can also become saggier and looser as we age, causing what is often referred too as "turkey neck" and "jowls". Excess fat can cause the jaw area to look less defined. For targeted solutions to these problems, there are some useful exercises in the "Face Yoga and You" chapter but the following five techniques are wonderful to help ease tension, improve skin quality and lift the jaw area.

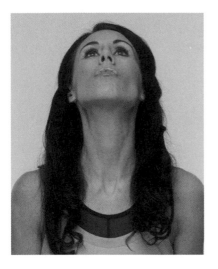

HOLD THE PUCKER

- - - -

1 Tilt your head back as far as is comfortable for you without straining your neck. Bring your lips into a "pout" position where your lips are pushed outward but not so they are squeezed in too tight that you are creating lines around the lips. Hold there for 30 seconds. Then open and close your mouth continuously for 30 seconds.

✳ **BENEFITS**
This helps to strengthen and tone many of the lower face muscles, which may lift and firm the attached skin.

✳ **TOP TIP**
Ensure you are opening the mouth equally on both sides by feeling the jaw area or checking in a mirror.

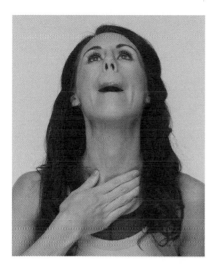

THE COLLAR BONE PRESS

----

1 Tilt your head back as far as is comfortable for you and wrap your lips around your teeth. Whilst maintaining this, bring your mouth into a smile shape, feeling the cheeks lifting. Place a hand onto your collarbone to act as resistance and encourage the muscles to work harder. Hold this position for 30 seconds. Take a break and repeat for another 30 seconds. If you notice any lines being created on your cheeks, take your hand off your collarbone and use a hand each side of your face to tighten the skin.

✳ BENEFITS

This technique is great for toning the jawline, neck and cheeks. With practice it may tone up loose skin under the jaw and lift skin on the neck.

✳ TOP TIP

Use "mind muscle" connection here. Focus on strengthening and toning the muscles. Your thoughts should be saying "strong yet relaxed".

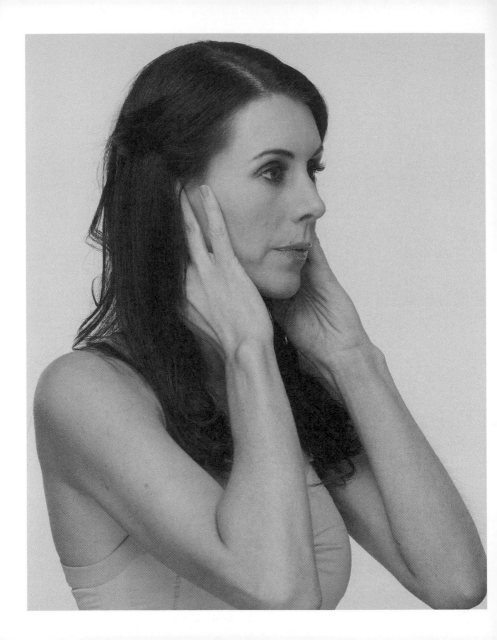

THE EAR COMB

----

1 Place your ring finger and little finger of both hands in front of your ears and the middle and index fingers behind your ears.

2 With gentle pressure, stroke the fingers downward, right down the neck. Do this for 1 minute.

❋ BENEFITS

This technique is great for draining excess lymph from the face, which can cause puffiness and dull skin tone, toward the lymph nodes in the collarbone. It is also a very nurturing and soothing massage to encourage your jaw area to feel more relaxed.

❋ TOP TIP

Very light touch is key here. The lymph vessels are located in the middle layer of skin, the dermis, which is closer to the surface than the fatty tissue and muscle. You don't want to press so hard that you feel the muscle. Use light, long downward strokes.

THE JAW TONER

----

1 Take your index finger, middle finger and thumb on both hands and gently pinch along your jaw line, toward your ears, pinching and releasing. Do this for 30 seconds, only ever moving upward.

2 Then, take your thumbs and place them next to each other on the chin at the jaw line. Stroke them along the jaw, away from each other. Lift them off when you reach the ears and start again. Do this for 30 seconds.

✱ BENEFITS

This is an excellent exercise for releasing and preventing jaw tension and may reduce jaw pain and teeth grinding that can come from stress. It also helps to improve the blood flow to your muscles, which will help the jaw to look and feel more lifted and firm.

✱ TOP TIP

Try to pinch down into the muscle so you stimulate all three layers of skin rather than just pulling up the top layer of skin. As you stroke along the jaw, try to allow the fingers to glide; a small drop of plant-based serum can aid with this.

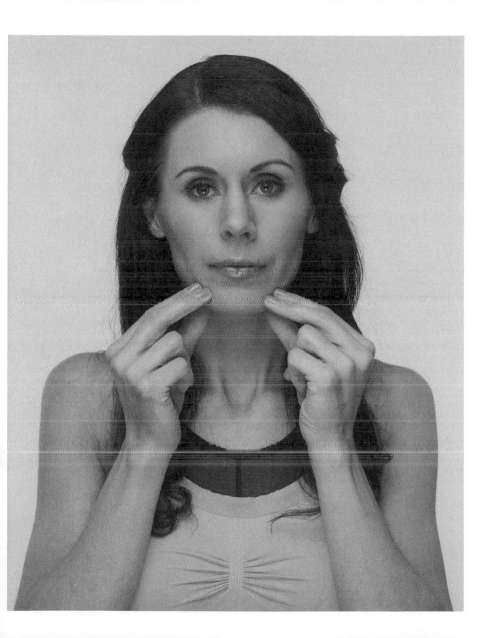

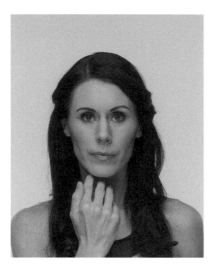

CHIN FINGER WIGGLE

----

1 Using the tops of your index, middle and ring fingers on one hand, tap under the chin area, working all the way up to one ear lobe and back across in the other direction. Continue for 1 minute, ensuring the rest of the face is relaxed.

✳ BENEFITS
This helps to brighten your skin by improving circulation and also helps to firm the muscles under the jaw.

✳ TOP TIP
If you want to get a gentle stretch in the neck and work the jaw area more, you can slightly tilt the head backward.

I AM FULL OF JOY

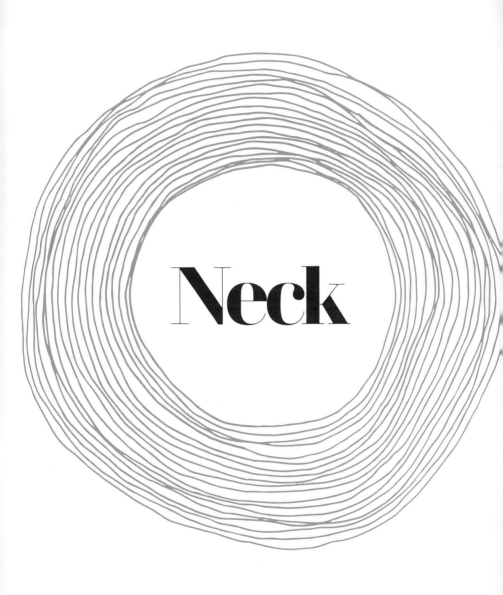

Neck

The neck area can age due to a number of reasons. A reduction in collagen and elastin can cause the muscles to loosen and get pulled downward by gravity. The constant downward gaze from repetitive phone use can cause lines and wrinkles. The thinner neck skin is also often forgotten when it comes to cleansing, toning moisturizing, exfoliating and SPF protection.

The neck is prone to tension. Reducing and preventing this tension may have direct relaxation and pain-relief benefits but it can also relieve tension in the rest of the face, which helps the face look more lifted. The neck area is home to key lymph nodes so it is an ideal place to do lymphatic drainage to help the skin on the face look brighter. In this chapter you will learn a basic lymphatic drainage technique, a shoulder release, a neck release, a neck-lifting technique and a neck massage technique.

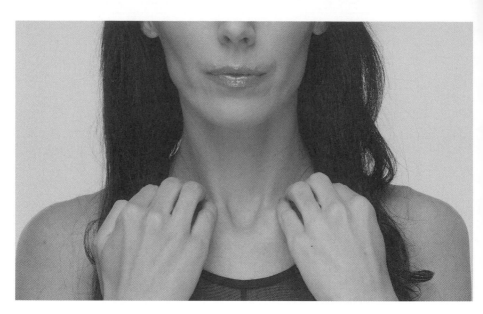

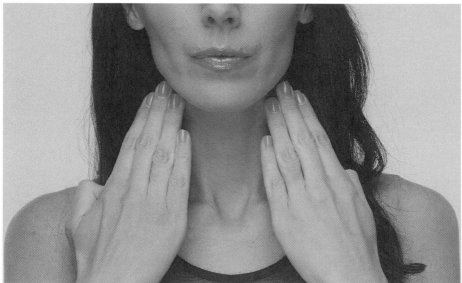

NECK LYMPHATIC DRAINAGE

----

1 Place the four fingers of both hands in the indent just above your collarbones. Press very lightly and then flick off. Do this pulsing massage at the rate of one pulse per second for 20 seconds.

2 Then place your fingers at the side of the neck, near the top. With a feather-like touch, stroke down the neck to the collarbone, being careful not to drag the skin. Lift the fingers off and come back to the starting position. Continue for 20 seconds.

3 Then repeat the first collarbone pulse again.

✳ BENEFITS

This helps to drain stagnant lymph, which means brighter skin, a less bloated face and a clearer complexion. It may also help clear the nose and throat and reduce swollen glands.

✳ TOP TIP

If you have time you could do up to 2 minutes of pulsing, then 2 minutes of stroking followed by 2 minutes of pulsing again. Lymphatic drainage works well done very gently with multiple repetitions. Remember, the lighter the touch, the better.

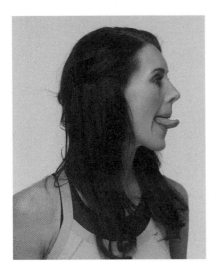

THE GECKO

----

1 Turn your head to one side and slightly tilt it back. Extend your tongue out as far as you can and hold for 15 seconds.

2 Gently turn your head to the other side and extend the tongue and hold for 15 seconds again. Repeat once more on both sides.

✳ BENEFITS
This helps to lift and firm the muscles on the side of the neck and jaw.

✳ TOP TIP
To further enhance the benefits of this exercise, point the chin up toward the ceiling a little more whilst the head is turned.

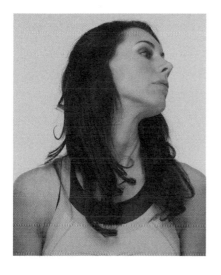

NECK ROLLS

----

1 Bring your chin down toward your chest and roll your chin from side to side, feeling a stretch in the back and sides of the neck. Continue for 30 seconds.

2 Do full circles with the neck, 3 times in one direction and 3 times in the other direction. It is essential that you only do what is comfortable for you, particularly if you have any neck issues.

✳ BENEFITS

This yoga technique can reduce and prevent neck tension, which can help you feel more comfortable and less stressed, and create a better posture.

✳ TOP TIP

To further release tightness in the back of the neck, slightly open the mouth.

THE NECK PINCH

- - - -

1 Using your index finger, ring finger and thumb of both hands, gently pinch the skin at the bottom of your neck, either side of your windpipe, feeling down to the muscle. Continue pinching gently up your neck. Move your hands a couple of centimetres (1 inch) away from each other and, starting at the bottom again, do the same thing, moving upward. Go back to your first position and continue this sequence for 1 minute in total.

✳ BENEFITS

This massage helps to firm and smooth the skin on your neck. As you pinch you encourage fresh blood, nutrients and oxygen up to the top layer of skin and aid the skin's ability to detoxify.

✳ TOP TIP

The pinches should be gentle but work right down to the muscle. So think pinching down rather than pulling the skin up. Remember how thin the skin is on the neck – we don't want to damage the skin.

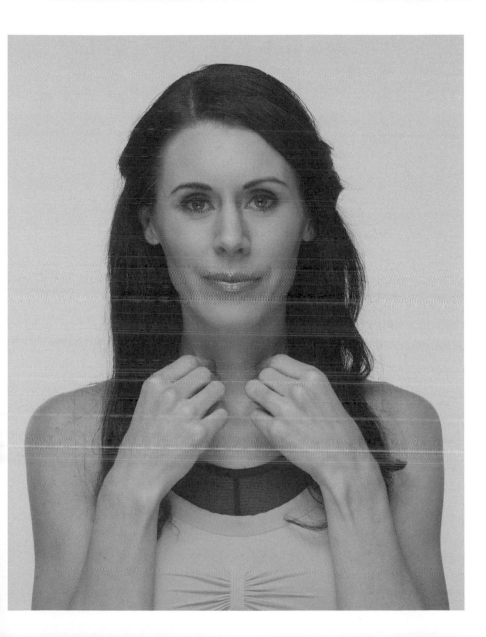

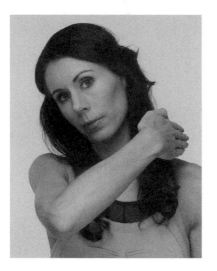

THE SHOULDER HACK

----

1 Tilt your head to the right so that your right ear comes toward your right shoulder. Using the edge of one hand, tap or "hack" the area where your neck meets your left shoulder for 20 seconds.

2 Use the same part of your hand to smooth down the shoulder for 10 seconds. Tilt the head to the left side and repeat.

✳ **BENEFITS**
This helps to ease tension in the shoulders and neck, and improves flexibility and posture in the area.

✳ **TOP TIP**
This works really nicely with a natural muscle-relaxing oil.

I AM
confident

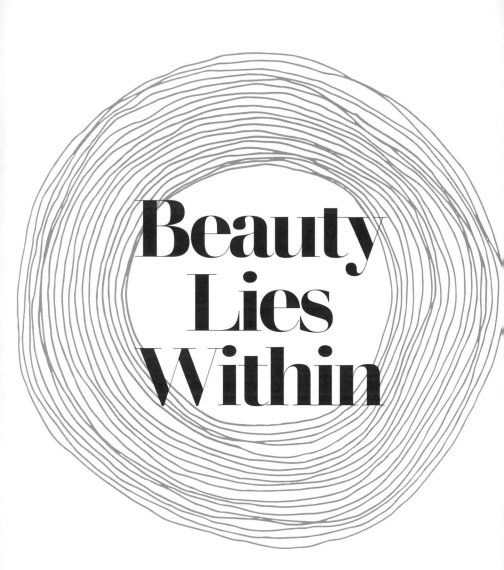

Exercise, massage, acupressure and relaxation are all incredibly important, but in order to get the aesthetic results you want, your lifestyle, including the food that you eat, your self-care routine and what is happening in the mind and body, plays a major role.

YOU ARE WHAT YOU EAT

What you eat is as important for your skin as your daily Face Yoga techniques. A healthy lifestyle can make the difference between glowing skin and dull, unhealthy skin. Moving toward eating more healthy natural foods and starting to reduce the unhealthy ones can support your goal of looking and feeling the best version of you.

FOODS TO AVOID

Refined sugar, alcohol and caffeine have been proven to age the face and can have negative effects on health overall. It is important to reduce fried, refined and processed food. We are all completely different, and for one person, foods like dairy, gluten and meat may not be beneficial for the skin or overall health, and for another person they may tolerate small amounts as part of a healthy, balanced diet. Don't cut out whole food groups without consulting a medical professional, and if you do decide that certain foods don't feed your skin, find other foods that contain the nutrients you may be missing.

QUENCH YOUR SKIN

In order to support your Face Yoga routine, water is key. Water has many benefits, such as aiding lymphatic drainage and circulation, which helps promote clearer, smoother skin. Water quenches dehydrated skin which means the skin is less dry and lines and wrinkles are therefore less apparent.

In the morning, fill up bottles with 2 to 3 litres (3½ to 5¼ pints) of water and drink throughout the day so you can measure how much you're having. The body better retains water when you sip it gradually, rather than drinking huge amounts in one sitting.

FOOD HEROES

Listed on the following pages are nourishing foods that can give you healthy glowing skin and help support your Face Yoga and your health in general. Incorporate a few of these foods into your diet and beauty regime every day for vibrant skin that is nourished inside and out.

BEST FOODS FOR SKIN HYDRATION:

Watermelon is the number one hydrating fruit due its 92 per cent water content. It also contains essential nutrients such as potassium, magnesium and sodium. Watermelons are high in vitamin C which is vital for collagen synthesis and the beta carotene and lycopene content works alongside your SPF to protect the skin from harmful rays.

Spinach is high in the antioxidant vitamin A which helps keep skin cells healthy and aids skin healing. The vitamin C content helps with collagen production and vitamin K helps strengthen blood vessels, which could reduce dark circles and inflamed skin.

Peaches are a great addition to your diet and can help the skin to look hydrated and firm. They have a water content of 89 per cent and are high in vitamin C which helps in the formation of collagen and fights free radical damage from toxins. Peaches also contain skin-friendly materials such as potassium and manganese.

Coconut water has been proven to restore hydration after exercise better than water due to its high content of electrolytes (salts and minerals that have lots of

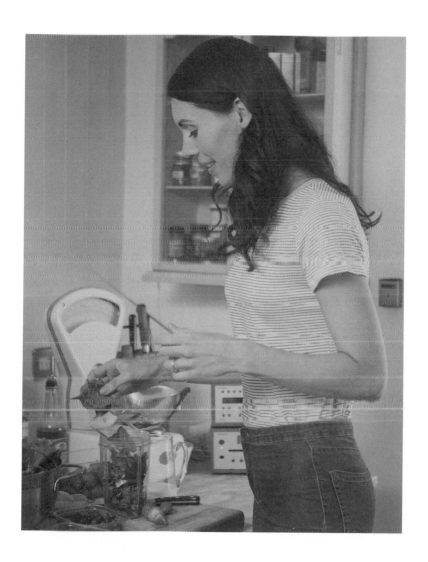

benefits, such as maintaining fluid balance). It is also high in antioxidants which protect cells from free radical damage.

Cucumber has the highest water content of any vegetable so is wonderful for the skin. Cucumber has long been famed for its ability to revitalize the skin around the eyes. I still haven't found a better food for topically cooling, hydrating and de- puffing the eye area.

BEST FOODS FOR SKIN LIFTING:

Lentils are a wonderful source of plant-based protein, which supports the muscles and collagen in the skin. Lentils are a nutritious and versatile addition to your diet. They are rich in vitamins and minerals, such as magnesium which helps reduce muscle tension, promotes sleep and supports the nervous system.

Quinoa contains 11 grams (1/3 ounce) of protein per cup and is rich in all 9 essential amino acids, making it one of my all-time favourite foods. It is gluten free, low GI, vegan, high in fibre and exceptionally high in vitamins and minerals.

Nuts are a wonderful source of omega 3, which has a number of benefits such as promoting skin firmness and reducing inflammation. Many varieties of nuts contain skin-healing vitamin A, E, zinc and selenium. Nuts are wonderful source of protein, with almonds being one of the highest at 30 grams (1 ounce) per cup.

Yogurt is an easy natural face mask to apply to the skin. It contains lactic acid which acts as a natural exfoliator for the skin due to its alpha hydroxyl acid content. Therefore it can help with the removal of dead skin cells, making the skin appear smoother and firmer. It also contains zinc and probiotics which have anti-inflammatory and healing and calming benefits.

Apply a thick layer, relax for 20 minutes and remove with warm water and a muslin cloth. Apply toner and then moisturiser.

BEST FOODS FOR GLOWING SKIN:

Tomatoes are high in lycopene which has been proven to help the skin build a defence against UV rays from the sun. Tomatoes are also rich in vitamin C and vitamin A, both of which are needed for healthy skin.

Berries are one of the fruits highest in antioxidants, so help to fight free radical damage in the skin. They are also high in ellagic acid and vitamin C which help to reduce and prevent skin damage. Studies have also shown that berries could block the production of the enzyme that breaks down collagen in the skin.

Carrots are a great source of vitamins A and C, both of which are important if you are prone to dry skin, eczema or acne. The carotenoids also have beneficial effects for healing skin wounds and for healthy eyes.

Avocados are high in vitamins A, C and E, potassium, essential fatty acids and lecithin, a fatty substance that can restore hydration in the skin. The oleic acid in avocados has been proven to have moisturizing and calming effects for dry and irritated skin.

Manuka Honey makes a nourishing face mask and multiple studies have highligted its benefits for clearing the skin and also for skin healing, treating acne and reducing inflammation. It has been noted for its hydrating properties which may have anti-ageing benefits. Apply to cleansed skin and leave for 15 minutes then remove with warm water and a muslin cloth.

BEST FOODS FOR SKIN CLEANSING:

Ginger contains gingerols, anti-inflammatory chemicals that have nourishing effects on the joints and the skin. Ginger is high in antioxidants which protect the face against ageing free radical damage.

Olives are high in vitamin E which protects the skin from UV radiation and pollutants. Olives and olive oil have skin-clearing benefits due to their anti-inflammatory properties.

Mushrooms are high in B vitamins which are important for energy and reducing stress levels as well as reducing inflammation. They contain polysaccharides for hydration, selenium and vitamin D for skin health and antioxidants for skin renewal and repair.

Kale is a powerhouse of nutrition for the face, body and mind. I recommend you eat it for healthy and glowing skin because of the balance between omega 3 and omega 9, which both have anti-inflammatory, lubricating and hydrating benefits. It is particulary high in vitamin K which benefits the bones. The very high antioxidant content makes it the ideal skin food.

LOVE YOURSELF

What is your first thought when you look in the mirror? Be truthful with yourself. Are you critical of the reflection looking back at you? If so, you certainly aren't alone. We can become convinced that the negative things we tell ourselves are reality rather than an opinion. This can have such a devastating effect on our wellbeing and health and can filter into every aspect of our day.

A helpful exercise to remedy this negativity and promote self-love is to create a "likes list". Simply write down ten things that you like, even love, about yourself, making sure that at least five of these are about your facial appearance. If you struggle to write a likes list, ask a friend, partner or family member to help you. Put the list somewhere you will see it every day.

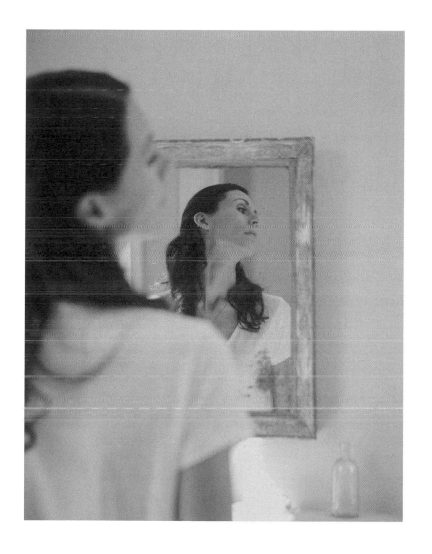

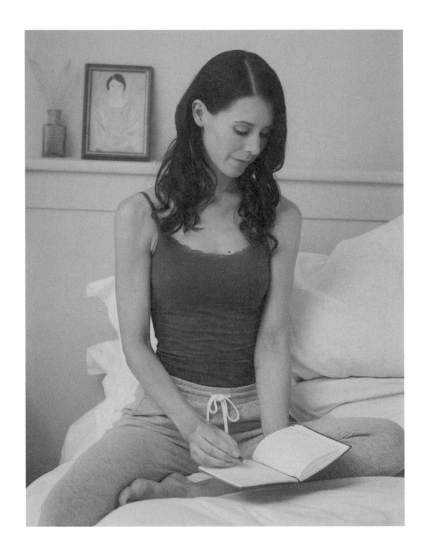

TAKE CARE

"I must look after myself." How does it feel to say those five words out loud? Maybe you think, yes, that's so important and I do lots of things to look after myself. Or maybe you instantly know that you don't look after yourself well enough or find yourself feeling guilty or selfish when doing things for you

I am here to say you MUST look after yourself. It isn't selfish, and you shouldn't feel guilty doing it. If you are someone who likes to look after others, though this is a wonderful quality, it's now time to make yourself a priority, too. You DESERVE to look and feel great. You are not only worthy of self-care but it is essential for living the healthiest, longest and happiest life.

TAKE A BREATH

If I had to pick only one wellbeing technique, it would be correct breathing. The word "correct" is key. Breathing happens every second of our life but we often breathe in a shallow, rapid way which can make us feel stressed.

Correct breathing has been proven to help the body and mind and when we have a healthy body and mind this positively impacts on the face. It also encourages mindfulness, which helps you to be in the present moment, reduces stress and boost health. Some of the proven benefits of doing regular deep breathing are:

1 Improved energy levels
2 Improved mood
3 Relaxation
4 Reduced anxiety and depression
5 Reduced pain and tension
6 Improved focus and concentration
7 Benefits for the heart
8 Reduced symptoms of stress-related illness
9 Reduced build-up of stress lines and wrinkles
10 Reduced inflammation.

HOW TO BREATHE PROPERLY

Start by noticing how you are breathing now by placing one hand on your chest and one hand on your abdomen. Which hand is moving more? If it's the hand on your chest then your breathing is probably too shallow and possibly too quick. You may also notice you are breathing mostly in and out through your mouth.

Gently close your lips and take a deep breath in through your nose, then slowly exhale through your nose. Continue with this until the breath is as slow as you can make it. Then let your abdomen rise with each in breath and fall with each out breath. Feel your belly and ribcage expand completely as you inhale and then the belly flatten and the ribcage soften on the exhale.

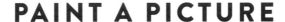

PAINT A PICTURE

Visualization is using your mind to imagine a situation, seeing every sight, sound and smell and feeling as though it is happening in the here and the now. It can aid in relaxation, goal achievement, concentration, motivation and even reduce anxiety and fear.

So how do you visualize? It is actually a very simple process.

Imagine your bed. Think about what colour it is, what material it is made out of. Think about the texture of the bed sheets. Think about how it feels to lay your head on the pillow and let your body sink in to the mattress. Think about the feel of the covers on your body, the scent of your bed and the temperature of the room. Are you experiencing this? If so, you are visualizing!

VISUALIZATION FOR GREAT SKIN

In your Face Yoga practice, the proven benefits of visualization can help you achieve your goal for great skin. At least once a week, sit or lie down and visualize yourself with the skin you want. See your face as smooth, lifted and firm. See your eyes as sparking and healthy. See your skin as glowing, vibrant and radiant. Visualize the areas you want to improve the way you would like them. If you find this easier to do by writing it down, drawing it or even looking in the mirror, then do that.

Now, sometimes you may find that negative emotions come up when doing this activity. You may find yourself saying that what you want isn't possible or that you can't achieve it. You may find it hard to see your face any way other than how it currently is. You may even be telling yourself that you are setting yourself up for failure or setting goals too high. Don't worry, visualize as much as you comfortably can, really trying to feel the way you would if you had the skin you want. Make these feelings stronger and stronger and more and more real. Remember that the true essence of The Danielle Collins Face Yoga Method is feeling great, so it's important to visualize this too.

GOOD POSTURE

Poor posture has been linked to everything from neck and back pain to headaches and sleep problems. All of this has an impact on the health of the face and the aesthetics of the skin. A 21st-century phenomenon is "tech neck", which is caused by increased cellphone and computer usage. This can result in lines and loose skin on the neck, tension in the jaw and tight muscles, which impede blood flow.

HOW TO IMPROVE YOUR POSTURE:

1   Bring your phone up in front of your face when typing rather than your head and neck down.
2   Use a hands-free phone.
3   Change your desk around so that your eyes are mid-screen height, your legs are at a 90 degree angle and your back is straight.
4   Improve your core strength through daily exercise and engage the lower tummy muscles to protect the lower back.
5   Do daily stretches for the neck, back, shoulders and hips to release tightness and tension.

BEAUTY SLEEP

Getting quality sleep is an essential part of your Face Yoga routine. Sleeping seven to nine hours a night helps your skin look its best. Visible signs you may notice from poor sleep are dark circles under the eyes, and thinner, drier and looser skin. Your face may also look duller, more blemished and more lined.

10 REASONS SLEEP HELPS OUR SKIN:

1. Collagen is made when you sleep.
2. Skin cells renew when you sleep.
3. Blood flow to the skin is boosted when you sleep.
4. Your skincare products work best when you sleep.
5. Your facial expressions are more relaxed after you have slept.
6. Your stress levels are lower when you sleep well.
7. Your skin eliminates toxins when you sleep.
8. Your skin isn't experiencing inflammatory fluctuations when you sleep.
9. There are fewer environmental free radicals when you sleep.
10. Your skin naturally exfoliates when you sleep.

HOW CAN WE GET A BETTER NIGHT'S SLEEP?

Turning all screens off two hours before bed is a good way to stop your mind being overactive before and while you sleep. The blue light emitted by computers, TVs and phones can negatively affect the internal body clock and not only make it harder to fall asleep but may also affect the quality of sleep.

Two to three drops of lavender oil on the pillow is a wonderful way to encourage your body and mind to feel relaxed and sleepy.

Going to bed and waking up at a regular time can support our internal body clock. We start to produce the sleep hormone melatonin around 9pm, so either go to sleep or start winding down around then.

Having a good bedroom environment can help to promote feelings of relaxation. Evidence shows that the ideal room temperature should be between 15 to 19 degrees Celsius (59 to 66 degrees Farenheight).

Reducing stimulants such as alcohol, caffeine and sugar before bed can help you get a better night's sleep. Many people feel alcohol helps promote sleep but in fact it can reduce the quality of your sleep and make it harder for the body to do its usual repair and renewal through the night.

Don't go to bed hungry. Ideally a small snack a couple of hours before bedtime means that your blood sugar levels won't drop too low in the early hours of the morning, which can wake you up. Equally try not to go to bed straight after a heavy meal because the body will be so busy trying to digest your food that it won't be able to do its usual repair and renewal routine.

Warm baths are a proven way to help promote better sleep. As we cool down afterwards and our body temperature drops, our body prepares for sleep. Our circadian rhythm is linked to temperature too.

There may be certain times in our lives when we struggle to get enough sleep. For me, it was the first year after having both my children. I was waking in the night for feeds and was often up early. I knew that there was nothing I could do about it and I just had to wait until they got a little older. Face Yoga really helped me during this time as I would use acupressure techniques and breathing exercises to help me get back to sleep after being awoken in the night. I also used Face Yoga to help my sleep-deprived skin look better in the morning.

YOGA

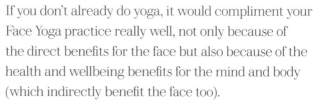

If you don't already do yoga, it would compliment your Face Yoga practice really well, not only because of the direct benefits for the face but also because of the health and wellbeing benefits for the mind and body (which indirectly benefit the face too).

Before starting a yoga practice, you must listen to your body and never do anything which causes pain or discomfort. If you have any medical conditions, please check with your doctor before starting. The techniques on the following pages are not intended to be a step-by-step guide to practice but instead an introduction on how certain types of poses can benefit you. For a full class, please visit an experienced qualified teacher, or you can use my yoga apps or DVDs.

I describe yoga as "cleaning out the tension" because after each practice I feel a such a shift in energy and a release of what is no longer serving me in mind, face and body. The moment I start any yoga practice, I feel a sense of being my true self. Whether you are new to yoga or an experienced practitioner, what I wish for you in your practice is the same: peace, mindfulness and contentment.

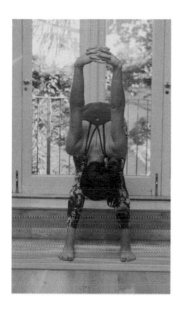

FORWARD BENDS

Forward bends are known in yoga as the calming poses. Multiple studies have shown that yoga may help reduce stress and anxiety as well as improving flexibility.

HOW THIS BENEFITS THE FACE

Forward bends are wonderful for encouraging fresh blood, oxygen and nutrients toward the face to nourish and brighten the skin. They also help release tension in the head, face and neck.

TOP TIP: Soften your knees in forward bends and always start by going to 80 per cent of what feels comfortable, not pushing it to your full capacity, to avoid back strain.

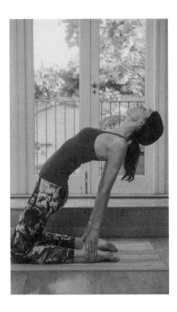

BACKBENDS

Back bends are known as
the energizing poses. They
are wonderful for balancing
out the hunched posture
that phones, sofas and
computers encourage".
The wonderful thing about
backbends is that they allow
the chest and lungs to fully
expand which encourages
deep abdominal breathing.

HOW THIS BENEFITS THE FACE

Back bends are great for
toning, lifting and firming the
front of the neck and jaw area.
They also release shoulder and
neck strain which can help to
reduce lines and loose skin on
the lower face.

.

TOP TIP: Fully warm up
before doing a back bend
and ensure your shoulders
are away from your ears.

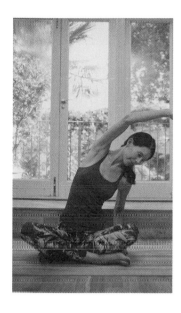

SIDE BENDS

I like to call side bends the "making space" poses. They help create more freedom and flow. After doing them you feel like you have created space to move better, think better and breathe better. Evidence shows that yoga may help to improve quality of life overall as well as reducing the secretion of the major stress hormone cortisol.

HOW THIS BENEFITS THE FACE

Side bends encourage the muscles in the side of the face and neck to engage, which can have a lifting effect. They also help to improve posture and reduce head and neck strain.

TOP TIP: One side of the body will always feel stronger and more flexible than the other, so use a full-length mirror to ensure you use both sides equally to readdress this natural imbalance within the body.

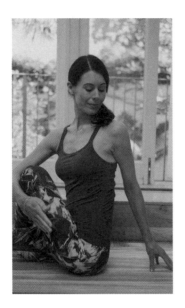

TWIST POSES

Although I'm not a fan of the word "detox"), twist poses can best be described as the detoxing poses because they gently aid the body's clever natural detoxification process. They help to improve circulation and boost the lymphatic system which may help with effective toxin removal. Evidence shows that twist poses can help to tone the vagus nerve, which is linked to our stress/ relaxation response.

TOP TIP: It is really common to lift the shoulders up to the ears, so take a moment to relax the shoulders and lengthen the neck.

HOW THIS BENEFITS THE FACE

Twist poses are really helpful for releasing tension in the neck and shoulders which in turn releases tension from the face. They also engage the muscles at the side of the face which has lifting and firming benefits.

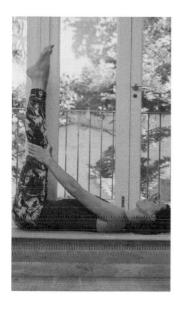

INVERSIONS

Inversions are known as the circulation poses. Inversions encourage better blood flow and studies show that they may reduce pain and have a positive effect on conditions such as depression.

HOW THIS BENEFITS THE FACE

Inversions are wonderful for bringing fresh blood and nutrients to the face, which helps to instantly brighten the skin and aids the removal of toxin build-up. Inversions also benefit the lymphatic system which helps reduce puffiness and dark circles under the eyes.

TOP TIP: If you have your period, are pregnant or have any medical conditions, it's best to avoid strong inversion poses.

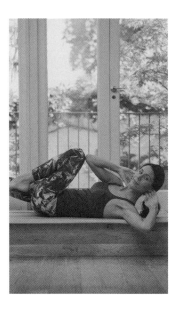

CORE POSES

Core poses are the strength poses. A strong core gives support to the rest of the body. Evidence shows that yoga can help build a strong core and also help build overall endurance.

HOW THIS BENEFITS THE FACE

Doing regular core strength helps to improve back, neck and shoulder health. This helps improve posture and release pain and strain, helping to prevent tightness in the jaw, neck and mouth area. Whilst doing core poses, ensure you're relaxing the jaw, and not pulling in the eyebrows or crinkling the forehead.

TOP TIP: Whilst doing core exercises, pull your lower abdominals up and in like you are zipping up a tight pair of jeans.

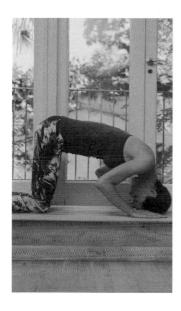

BALANCE POSES

Balance poses are known as the centering poses. Our balance literally comes from our centre (our core) but these poses also promote feeling of centeredness and focus. Evidence shows that balance poses promote mindfulness, which can have so many benefits for the mind, body and face.

HOW THIS BENEFITS THE FACE

Balance poses involve focusing on one point while fully relaxing the facial muscles. Being mindful of the face and learning to release and prevent tension is key to reducing expression lines.

TOP TIP: While holding your pose, open the eyes wide without raising the eyebrows to strengthen the eye muscles. Relax all other facial muscles. This will prevent tension lines building up.

A FINAL WORD

I hope this book has given motivation to use these simple and effective tips and techniques to look and feel the most wonderful version of you. Everything I share with you comes from years of personal and professional experience and passion. If you integrate this Method into your life I am certain you will glow inside and out. As a final word, just remember...

Do Face Yoga because you are proud of ageing, proud of who you are and proud that it's you putting the hard work in to get results. Do Face Yoga because each day you strive to love yourself a little more and want look and feel the best you can for your age. Do Face Yoga to have an amazing tool kit for glowing skin, a healthy body and a happy mind. Do Face Yoga because it nourishes your soul as well as your face.

Wishing you lots of love and light,
Danielle xx